DANIÈLE RYMAN'S

Secrets

of youth & beauty

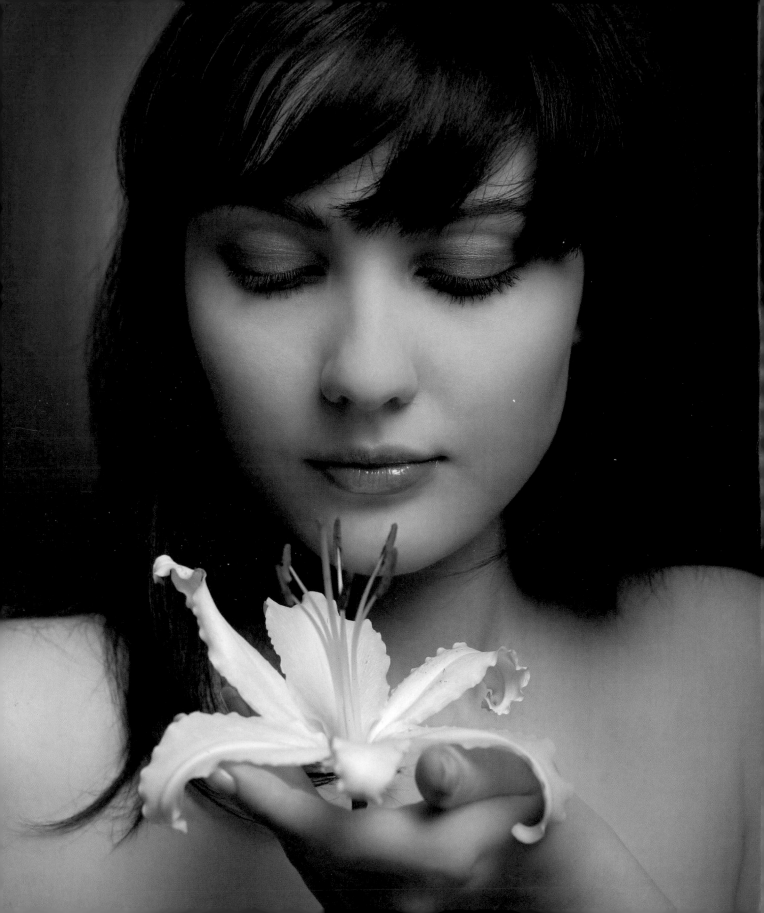

DANIÈLE RYMAN'S

Secrets

of youth & beauty

aromatherapy for natural rejuvenation

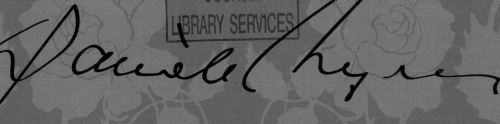

RODALE®

MACMILLAN

First published in 2007 by Rodale Ltd
an imprint of Pan Macmillan Ltd
Pan Macmillan, 20 New Wharf Road, London N1 9RR
Basingstoke and Oxford
Associated companies throughout the world
www.panmacmillan.com

ISBN: 978-1-905744-06-0

Copyright ©2007 Danièle Ryman

Illustrations by Ray Smith/CIA
Edited by Carol Franklin
Designed by Briony Hartley/Goldust Design
Picture research by Dawn Bates
Managing editor Anne Lawrance

1 3 5 7 9 8 6 4 2

A CIP record for this book is available from the British Library

Printed and bound in Singapore by Star Standard

Notice: This book is intended as a reference volume only, not as a medical manual. The
information given here is designed to help you make informed decisions about your health.
It is not intended as a substitute for any treatment that you may have been prescribed by your
doctor. Neither the author nor publisher shall be liable for any loss or injury arising as a result
of information in this book. If you suspect you have a medical problem, we urge you
to seek competent medical help.

Picture credits PRELIMS: **viii** Robin Matthews. **iStockphoto ii** Alexandr Denisenko; **vi** Ye Liew;
5 Christian Michael; **6** Rebecca Picard; **7** Daniel Gilbey; **12** Zsolt Nyulaszi PART ONE: **iStockphoto**
24 Tim Starkey; **26** Christopher Walker; **31** Slobo Mitic; **35** Gemma Ivern; **36** Douglas Freer; **40** Lisa
Mory; **43** Liv Friis-Larsen; **47** Monika Adamczyk; **48** Gaffera; **51** Pixonaut; **53, 58** Kelly Cline;
57 Elena Kalistratova; **60** Greg Nicholas; **66** Brandon Laufenberg. **Alamy 17** CuboImages srl; **20** Look
Die Bildagentur der Fotografen GmbH; **23** Konrad Zelazowski; **54** Foodfolio; **55** Rstudio; **62** Andrea
Jones; **67** Photo Resource Hawaii PART TWO: **73, 74** Stockbyte/Getty Images. **iStockphoto**
70 Matthew Bowden; **81** Iryna Shpulak; **83, 130** Liv Friis-Larsen; **100, 113** Kateryna
Govorushchenko; **103** Cristian Ardelean; **107** A E Knost; **112** Yanik Chauvin; **115** Jim DeLillo;
137 Leigh Schindler. **Alamy 95** Mark Scott; **124** Goodshoot Jupiterimages/France. PART THREE:
iStockphoto 140 Christian Michael; **146** Nikolay Suslov; **147** Fredrik Larsson; **152** Paul Piebinga;
158 Willie B. Thomas. **Alamy 163** Stockimage/Pixland

Visit **www.panmacmillan.com** to read more about all our books and to buy them. You will
also find features, author interviews and news of any author events, and you can sign up for
e-newsletters so that you're always first to hear about our new releases.

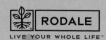

RODALE
LIVE YOUR WHOLE LIFE™

We inspire and enable people to improve their lives and the world around them

A Isabelle,
mon amie de toujours

Acknowledgements

I would like to thank the following people:

My god daughter and assistant, Natasha Kahn, for being so thoughtful in helping me organize my work and for devoting so much of her time to reading and deciphering my handwritten manuscript. We have been such a good team.

My editor Anne Lawrance, who was so patient, giving me time to complete this enjoyable task and working tirelessly to bring the text to completion.

Barbara Brittingham, my little sister and friend who always had good suggestions and ideas for my work.

My agents Pat Lomax and Eddie Bell, who supported my ideas for a new book from the start, and a great thank you to Pat who stimulated my thoughts during our catch-up lunches, saying 'You can do it'.

Sue Mousley, a special caring midwife from the George Eliot Hospital, for her unfailing help and kindness to get me information on essential oils she uses in the Maternity wards and for permission to reproduce her recipe for pregnancy massage oil.

A Caroline Colliard qui fut toujours une source d'inspiration.

And finally my family and in particular my husband James, who also encouraged me to write this book and has been such a great support in all my activities and who nurtures me with love and affection at every moment.

Un grand merci à ma petite mère, pour son amour et ses connaissances qui ont inspirés les recettes de certaines formules.

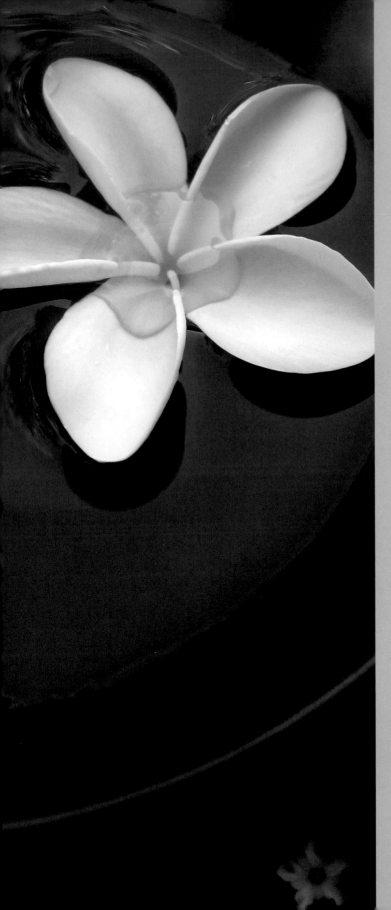

Contents

Part Two
FACE AND BODY BEAUTY AND ANTI-AGEING TREATMENTS

Part Three
PAMPERING

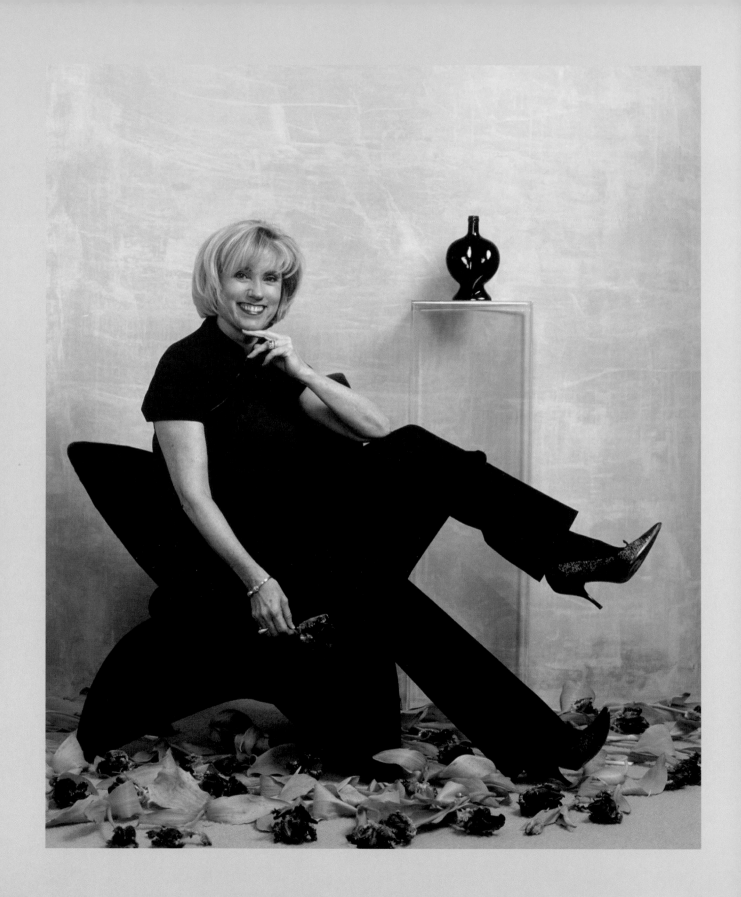

Introduction

After 40 years practising aromatherapy and writing books on the subject, I feel I have many solutions to the stressors of everyday life through the use of essential oils. This book offers 'my personal secrets' of health and beauty, which include the know-how to slow down the ageing process using essential oils and other natural ingredients. It is a refreshingly simple approach, combining Eastern and Western traditions, together with common sense and a passion and commitment to the power of nature.

It is through travelling the world many times, and living in many countries, seeking out ingredients and therapies, and my boundless curiosity and enthusiasm, together with my practical experience in the use of plants and natural ingredients, that my research has developed. Also, as a practitioner it has been valuable to observe the way people react to and use the world around them.

Health and beauty books are often written by journalists who are offering personal opinions based on research into their subject. It would be true to say that many such writers are not themselves practitioners. As a practitioner myself, I am able to give a totally different perspective, being able to draw my ideas and solutions from practical experience of the problems encountered by my patients, who have often spent large sums of money on conventional beauty products and treatments, with disappointing results. More and more, my patients are questioning what is safe in the cosmetics industry and why today's miracle product so often becomes tomorrow's scare story.

Not only is aromatherapy my subject but it is also my way of life and has helped me in so many difficult circumstances. It has given me the chance in a pleasant, aromatic way to cope with and thrive in many difficult situations throughout my life. I would like you to benefit from my experiences and to regain confidence in using the essences of nature to deal with your own ageing process in a more natural way. Also I would like to encourage you to follow my easy recipes and formulate and develop new regimes to help your appearance and health, and reduce stress. I believe passionately that everyone can have beautiful skin and that they should not need a bank loan to get it. Instead try a simple approach, using the best, most effective natural ingredients.

My secrets for health and beauty came from ancient civilizations where chemicals were not used and where working with nature was part of their everyday life. My family comes from the Lot in the Ardeche region of France, where nature has always been well respected. My grandparents were the first to initiate me into the family secrets and recipes passed down from generation to generation, using healing plants, flowers, seed, grains, floral waters, honey, vinegars, wines, tisanes, fruits and vegetables.

Aromatherapy is an ancient art and its history is lost in the mists of time. Archaeological excavations have uncovered signs of the use of medicinal herbs as long as 6000 to 9000 years ago. By the nineteenth century herbs and essential oils were being investigated scientifically to explain their usefulness in many areas of cosmetics and medicine, but aromatherapy was officially recognized in 1920 when René Gattefossé, a French chemist who became known as the Father of Aromatherapy, coined the name. After being badly burnt in his laboratory, his hand became infected, so he decided to test out the reputed pain-relieving properties of lavender oil. To his great surprise, Gattefossé found that lavender not only relieved the pain but also helped with healing and cured the infection. This encouraged him to research further into the applications of essential oils on the skin and also into their medicinal uses.

One of the most famous practitioners of aromatherapy was Dr Jean Valnet who used essential oils on wounded soldiers and civilians in the Second World War, owing to shortages of orthodox medicine. He has written many valuable books on the healing properties of essential oils based on his research.

One of the most prominent researchers in the cosmetics industry was Austrian-born Marguerite Maury, who was based in Paris and became known as the doyenne of aromatherapy. She developed a great reputation in France for her 'medico-cosmetic' therapy and was a firm believer in rejuvenation of the skin with essential oils. She carried out extensive research on the therapeutic benefits of essential oils, recognizing the potential of essential oils absorbed into the body through the skin. She found that essential oils encouraged the production of skin cells, refining wrinkles and keeping a youthful appearance, slowing the ageing process. She also noted the healing effect that essential oils had on internal organs and muscles and advised applying them every day. I had the privilege to study under Marguerite Maury, who was a charismatic, extraordinary woman, and I became her protégée and wanted to carry on her work after her death.

Marguerite Maury gave me my first prescription when I complained of a little wrinkle appearing round my eye at the age of 22. She made me a special oil, for which I still have the recipe: geranium, neroli, eucalyptus, rose, mixed in a carrier oil of avocado, hazelnut and almond. It smelt beautiful and was so effective that from that moment I was hooked.

There have been many years of research into the traditional uses of aromatic substances for beauty and rejuvenation and in recent years modern technology has permitted research into new ingredients designed to help slow the ageing process and beautify the skin. Women are spending more and more money on their faces and bodies and are very often disappointed by the results when they may actually be using the wrong beauty products. In fact many problems with ageing skin are made worse by our twenty-first-century lifestyle: fast food, stress, lack of exercise and industrial pollutants.

I hope that I will be able to pass on my passion and enthusiasm to you to enable you to use essential oils as I do everyday in my life. For example, they find a place in my home:

In my study, to help me to concentrate:
basil, jasmine, rose.

In my living areas, positive and cheerful smells:
eucalyptus, cedarwood, orange, lemon.

In my kitchen, for cleaning surfaces:
thyme, rosemary, lemon.

In the bedroom, to ensure a good night's sleep, I vaporize: *neroli, lavender, melissa.*

All essential oils, apart from their antiseptic and bactericide properties, have natural hormones and traces of vitamins, minerals and the antioxidants that are so important in rejuvenation. In this book you will learn how to recognize which oils are most suitable for your skin type and how to care for it most effectively. You will also be pleased to know that you will save money by making your own skin-care range and remedies and you will help look after the environment as well as your own health, since you will be using no synthetic chemicals, which can contaminate waterways.

Some essential oils have hit the headlines too. Research done in the USA on a small group of three young boys appeared to show that after topical application of tea tree and lavender oils their oestrogenic properties seemed to trigger the growth of breast tissue, a rare condition known as gynaecomastia, which often has no obvious cause. It would be interesting to know what other products they used. What were the synthetics or chemicals in the products? What was the diet of those three young boys? The product used in the research was a lavender-scented soap and it is not clear whether this contained true essential oil or a synthetic lavender fragrance. Later research on those two essential oils indicated that they actually possess weak oestrogenic properties. The situation currently is very confusing and more up-to-date findings are awaited.

It is important to realize that anyone can be allergic to anything natural, but most allergic reactions come from synthetic cosmetic ingredients. Follow the instructions for the recipes in this book carefully and do test patches and you should find you have no problems. You will have great fun concocting your own natural perfumes without the use of benzene derivatives and other toxins often found in commercial preparations, which can be harmful to health.

It is just as important to ask whether the ingredients of the products we use every day are safe. One cosmetic scientist, Judi Beerling, has stated that man-made chemicals are inherently dangerous, as the source of such chemicals tells you nothing about their safety. Here are some ingredients you may find in your cosmetics and every-day toiletries that should ring alarm bells:

Petrochemicals – can cause irritation and skin allergies.

Synthetic chemicals not found in nature (xenobiotics).

Solvent extracts (isolates).

Surfactants (sodium laureth and sodium lauryl sulphate have received recent negative publicity – research published in the medical journal *The Lancet* shows that lauryl sulphate can damage the barrier function of the skin, making it more susceptible to allergens).

L-menthol (synthetically produced, rather than extracted from the mint plant).

Synthetic fragrances – a major source of skin irritation in cosmetic products.

Parabens (preservatives claiming to have 'nature identical' properties, which are now under increasing suspicion).

Emulsifiers.

Sunscreens – usually contain parabens.

Colourants (which are an unnecessary additive).

The list is long! Natural alternatives do exist, for example lecithin from soya or casein from milk can both be used as emulsifiers.

It should also be appreciated that synthetic chemicals in beauty products are not only potentially harmful to our health but also to our environment and wildlife.

My conclusion is that we can't divorce from Nature as Nature is part of Life. And I hope through this book to show you that aromatherapy offers a natural way to stay and keep healthy and will enable you to feel and look more alive, vital and youthful. I wish you well as you explore its benefits for yourself.

Danièle Ryman

May 2007

Basics of aromatherapy

What are essential oils?

Essential oils are made up from a combination of different organic molecules, which give each oil its unique character. They are the plant's energy or soul and are found in flowers, seeds, bark, grains, roots and resins, as well as leaves, in minute quantities. They are found in both wild and cultivated plants and are responsible for the plant's aroma as well as being its main defence against infections and infestations. These molecules also help the growth and fertilization of the plant. As a US researcher, Dr Gary Young, stated in 1995, 'the essential oils in plants are what blood is to the human body, and much, much more'.

There are approximately 30,000 known aromatic molecules that make up the various essential oils and we have only begun to scratch the surface in identifying and making references about each of them. For instance, a simple essential oil such as sage contains up to 800 different chemical constituents and there are over 650 different varieties of sage! That is why, with the wonders of modern technology, we are continually able to discover new constituents and, with them, find new oils to be used in therapy.

Sometimes several different essential oils can be extracted from the same plant – the orange tree for example. The essential oil of orange comes from the zest of the fruit, petit grain is found in the leaves, and essential oil of neroli, with its wonderful scent, comes from the orange flowers. These oils have a few similar notes, but each has its own identity and therapeutic value.

There are approximately 300 different essential oils

There are approximately 300 different essential oils being utilized in aromatherapy — they are recognized by professional practitioners for their importance in healing.

being utilized in aromatherapy – they are recognized by professional practitioners for their importance in healing. For this book I have selected those that are in most common use as they can be bought easily and have been used in therapy for years. Each oil has its own identity, history, provenance, texture and qualities. Every essential oil varies in colour – some chamomiles, for instance, are yellow while others are blue. Both types are slightly different in their application and strength. Lavender is light and transparent, while patchouli and vetiver are thick and dark. The different aroma of each oil depends on its balance, as does its therapeutic value.

Even if you only used six out of the 300 essential oils distilled today, you would benefit greatly. If that seems a lot, two are a good start, as they will enable you to make a few therapeutic preparations. You need the synergy of two essential oils to reinforce and complement each other; for example, if you want to relax try lavender and petit grain because their calming, slightly hypnotic properties are strengthened when combined. Two, three or four essential oils will create a strong chemical structure when mixed together and some blends can become quite powerful – certain essential oils, such as peppermint, for example, act as amplifiers so you will find that I have used it sparingly in the recipes.

Principal extraction methods
Steam distillation

Most essential oils are extracted by steam. Applied heat and pressure release the essential oil in drops above a container. This process can be used to extract oils such as rose, geranium, eucalyptus, basil, peppermint etc. As the oil is lighter than water, it floats on the surface of the recipient before being separated. The water that remains is called hydrolat and is very aromatic. It is used in many cosmetic products or can be used on its own as, say, a toner or for medicinal purposes (rosewater and peppermint water for example). Approximately 5 tonnes

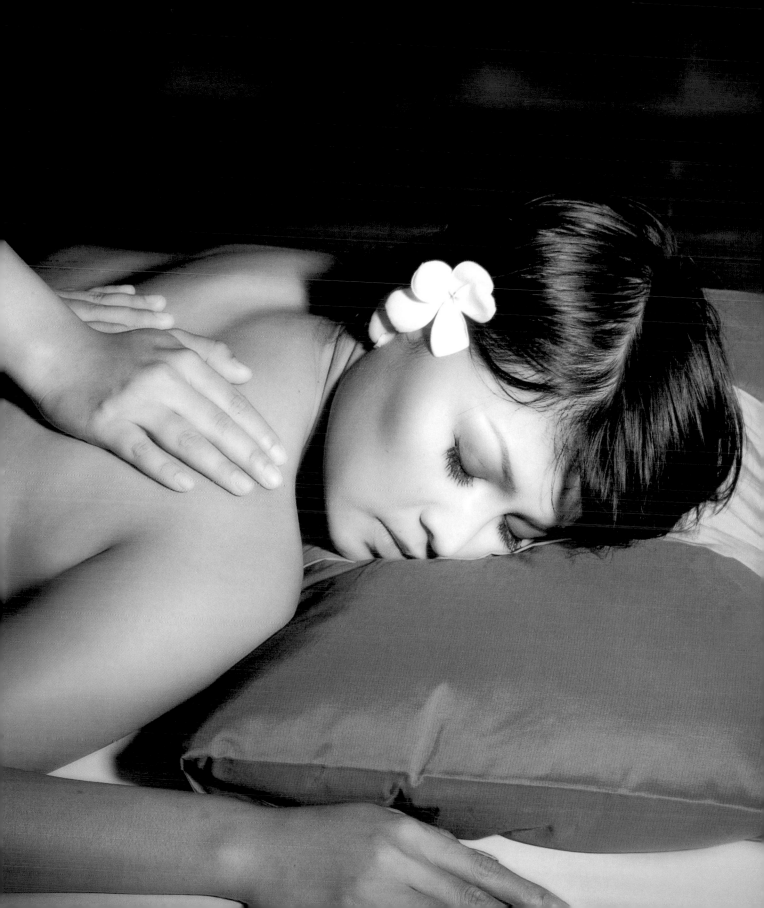

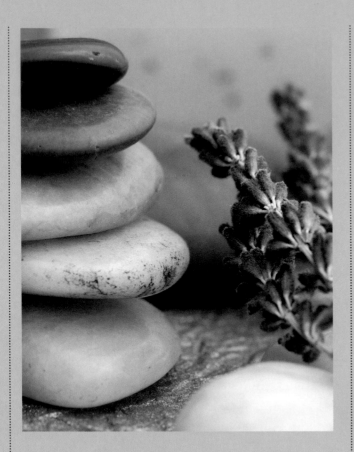

The constituents of essential oils

The primary elements of all essential oils are hydrogen, carbon and oxygen. However, they are also made up of hundreds of different components, the most common being terpenes, terpinols, alcohols, esters, aldehydes, ketones and phenols. The large number of these constituents makes it almost impossible to reproduce an oil synthetically. It is the constituents that give the essential oil its therapeutic value and unique qualities, and therefore imitations will never have the same power to treat, heal and rejuvenate.

Because of their chemical structure, essential oils are able to penetrate the epidermis, the membrane of the human cells, just as they do the cells of plants, to bring important nutrients inside. They reinforce the immune system, assisting with repair and healing, and strengthening its resistance to exterior attacks.

The particular qualities of the main constituents of essential oils are as follows:

Terpenes – these help the body get rid of accumulated toxins. They are antiseptic, anti-inflammatory, anti-viral and analgesic. They also have sedative properties.
Alcohols – these are anti-viral, anti-bacterial and anti-inflammatory. Linalool is one of the most important constituents in alcohol as it is highly anti-bacterial and is said to boost the immune system.
Aldehydes – these are anti-viral, antiseptic and have sedative properties. They are found in citrus oils.
Ketones – these are known to be good for cell rejuvenation as they promote the formation of tissue. They help to dissolve mucus and assist in its discharge.
Phenols – these kill bacteria and have powerful anti-oxidant properties, benefitting the immune system.

Using this book

I hope you will enjoy reading about the essential oils in this book. You will learn something about their history and therapeutic value – you will notice that most are antiseptics and some are considered to be natural antibiotics. (This is because they contain alcohol and terpenes.)

of roses are needed for 1kg (2¼lb) of rose essential oil – so just one drop represents a few kilograms of rose petals!

Expression

This technique is used to obtain the essential oils from the rind of fruits such as grapefruit, oranges, lemons and limes. The rinds can be grated or pressed and the oil from the torn cells is collected using a sponge. This used to be done by hand but the process is now mechanized.

Dissolving

This method of extracting oils involves volatile solvents. These are heated in a huge tank like a pressure cooker and the resulting substance is known as a 'concrete'. This is treated with alcohol that is then evaporated to leave behind a sticky substance. A concrete doesn't have the same therapeutic value as pure essential oil since chemical residues are often present. It is used mostly in the perfume industry.

Each of the oils I have chosen for this book comes with an explanation – their history, origin, properties and usage. Many have abilities to heal, rejuvenate, calm and relax, and you will see what they can do instantly. I have described the best way to use them to get the best results. For instance, you will discover that lavender is not the only essential oil to induce sleep, there are many others; and that myrrh was used and recorded by Ancient Egyptians as an effective antiseptic and as a healer of wounds and scars.

You will see that many essential oils are similar in their usage and because many of us don't always react in the same way, you will be able to find one that works for you. For example, lavender is classified as a calmer, but it could be a stimulant for some people, so you will need to identify what each oil does for you. You might also note that if your health changes, some oils may not work so well. Also, after using particular oils for a while your body may become accustomed to those oils and begin not to respond so well to them, so you may decide you want to try others. Revise your remedies and where options are given, change your formulations every couple of months.

You will find many interesting recipes to rejuvenate the skin in Parts Two and Three. You will save a lot of money by creating your own products and you will be able to adjust each recipe to suit you, getting the full benefit without any chemicals, preservatives or emulsifiers.

In this book you will find out that you can use essential oils in many different ways – as a vapour in your bedroom or office to help you calm down or to boost your energy for instance. I have detailed the safe oils to use during pregnancy and the best ways to use them. You will not only discover how to make your own perfume to suit your mood and create your individual identity, but also the best way to combat cellulite and how to enhance your exercise time. There are essential oils to help prepare the skin before and after cosmetic surgery and oils to help during the menstrual cycle and at menopause. You will find out the best oils to take with you on holiday and those that can uplift your mood and increase your passion! There are even oils that can be used as household antiseptics and air fresheners.

What you need to know

Essential oils are volatile molecules so can evaporate quickly. For example, if you spray your kitchen, in ten minutes the aroma will be in your bedroom. To slow down this volatility you need a carrier oil to trap the molecules and make the aroma diffuse slowly. If applying an essential oil to the skin, it is better to combine it with a carrier oil, in fact don't apply it neat unless directed. Particular care should be taken when using essential oils on older people, pregnant women or children. Always consult an expert. Some people may have allergic reactions so if you are sensitive, have had a problem in the past or are pregnant, always do a skin patch test first (see overleaf). And remember that essential oils should *never* be taken internally.

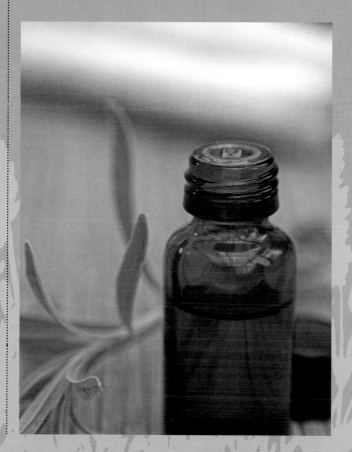

Skin patch test

❧ *People with sensitive skins and pregnant women should always do a skin patch test before they use essential oils for the first time. This is also recommended for anyone who suffers from hay fever or other allergies, and elderly people and children.*

Dip a cotton bud in a tiny trace of the essential oil and rub on the inside of your wrist – just gently touch the skin (you could also do this on the inside of the elbow or on the underside of the arm). Cover the area with a plaster and leave unwashed for twenty-four hours. After this time check for any redness, irritation or small spots. If you have even the tiniest reaction, do not use the oil. **Note:** *It is always worth trying again after a month as your skin may now accept the oil.*

Buying oils

Choose your essential oils and carrier oils carefully – they are all easily available in health shops and large supermarkets. When you purchase an essential oil, always check the expiry date, check the provenance and, most importantly, the Latin name on the label – make sure you buy the right variety as different varieties may have different properties. Always buy from a reputable shop as oils can often be adulterated and falsified. Don't be afraid to ask questions. Always sniff first – avoid oils that have lingering, pungent aromas. If you can afford to buy organic oils, do. These versions can be more potent and should be totally free from any impurity. I would particularly recommend them for times of illness, pregnancy or for skin problems. Finally, make sure the bottle is dark (exposure to light can affect the chemistry of the oil) and the cap is secure and tight.

Carrier oils

I have named many different carrier oils in the remedies in this book because they all have such different properties – some are better on the face, others on the body or in the bath (see chart opposite). All have excellent solvent qualities allowing the molecules in the essential oils to expand, giving their full-strength aroma (the carrier oils themselves should have little or no smell). These carrier oils have all given me satisfaction and good results over the years and are also readily available. You will also notice that I have included wheat-germ (vitamin E) capsules in many of the preparations. The capsules stop the oils from going rancid, but you should of course make sure you check the expiry date on the carrier oils. Don't use mineral oil – this is not good for the skin.

Gels and pastes

These can be made up easily and they really help revitalize the skin.

Pectin – this slightly acidic powder can be found in health food shops and large supermarkets. It has astringent qualities, closing pores and refining the skin. It is excellent mixed with essential oils. In general you need about 1 tablespoon of powder to 200ml (7 fl oz) of water. Follow instructions on packet and in recipes.

Slippery elm powder – this makes a wonderful base for masks as it soothes and hydrates the skin. It is easy to make too – just add a little cold water to two generous teaspoons of slippery elm powder to make a paste. Add a further 100–200ml (3$\frac{1}{2}$–7fl oz) of boiled water very slowly to make a looser paste. Simmer for twenty to twenty-five minutes. As the gel cools, it will thicken.

Natural toners for use in beauty preparations

Aloe vera juice – excellent to mix with essential oils, good for rehydration as it repairs and rejuvenates the skin. Helps healing and is a good natural moisturizer.

Black tea – slightly astringent, helps to maintain the colour of a tan.

Chamomile infusion – soothing, helps irritated and swollen skin.

Carrier oils

Name	Colour/ Consistency	Obtained	Contains	Usage
Almond oil (*Prunus amygdalus var. dulcis*)	very pale yellow; fluid	from the kernel	traces of vitamins and minerals	all skins, especially dry, wrinkled and sensitive. Good for inflamed or irritated, dehydrated and ageing skin. Softening action.
Argan oil (*Argania spinosa*)	pale yellow; thick	from the kernel	rich in vitamins, linolenic acid, powerful anti-oxidant	soothing and naturally antiseptic. Excellent oil for beauty use; accelerates healing of scar tissue and rejuvenation of the skin.
Avocado oil (*Persea americana*)	dark green; fluid	from the fruit	fatty acids, lecithin, traces of vitamins and proteins	very, very dry skins and those that lack tone and firmness. Good for dehydrated skin, wrinkles or people with psoriasis or eczema.
Borage oil (*Borago officinalis* or *Echium amoenum*) Also known as starflower	pale yellow; fluid	from the seeds	traces of vitamins and minerals and linolenic acid	reinforces the effects of other oils, increasing their benefits. Good for psoriasis and eczema, those with sensitive skin, too much sun and premature ageing. An excellent oil to rejuvenate skin tissue – helps with healing after surgery.
Castor oil (*Ricinus communis*)	colourless; thick, very viscous	from the seeds	fatty acids, ricinoleic acid and glycerine	good mixed with other carrier oils, nourishes the skin, rehydrates and helps to keep suppleness and softness.
Evening primrose oil (*Oenothera*)	very pale yellow; fluid	from seeds	traces of minerals and vitamins, gammalinolenic acid which helps the skin to retain moisture	good for menstrual problems (as anti-inflammatory properties relieve cramps and aches), eczema, dermatitis and psoriasis. Too much sun, anti-ageing. Reinforces the properties of other oils.

(continued)

Name	Colour/ Consistency	Obtained	Contains	Usage
Grapeseed oil (*Vitis vinifera*)	very slightly green, almost colourless; fluid	from the pips	traces of minerals, vitamins and proteins; high in polyunsaturates	good for all skin types, but especially oily skins. Can be used in conjunction with other oils. It is very fluid and light and is good in formulations for body oils, massage and facial serums (excellent for micro-circulation – circulation of the small capillaries).
Jojoba oil (*Simondsia chinensis*)	pale yellow; waxy	from the grain	ester of liquid wax, similar to human skin secretions (sebum)	good for all skin types, protects and gives a fresh and healthy look. Helps eliminate toxins and dirt. A good base for essential oils, used in perfume, body oils and bath products.
Rose masqueta oil (*Rosa officinalis*)	reddish-yellow; viscous	from the seeds	traces of vitamins and minerals	is uplifting, with excellent anti-ageing properties. Good in pregnancy and in treatment of stretchmarks, after plastic surgery.
Sesame oil (*Sesamum indicum*)	pale yellow; fluid	from the seeds	traces of proteins, minerals, vitamin B, lecithin, amino acids, anti-oxidants	excellent for all types of skin. Good after sun and for skin irritations such as eczema.
Soya oil (*Glycine hispida* or *soja*)	very pale yellow; fluid	from the beans	traces of vitamins, minerals and proteins	all skin types but especially oily skins, as it is slightly astringent and nourishing at the same time. Mixes well with other oils. Particularly good for massage.
Wheatgerm oil (*Triticum vulgare*)	a lovely yellow-orange; thick	from the germ of the wheat	high proportions of vitamin E and other vitamins, minerals and protein	good for counteracting premature ageing of the skin, dehydrated skin but all skin types will benefit. Prevents other oils from turning rancid, reinforces their properties. Good after cosmetic surgery.

Cider/wine vinegar – these are widely used in aromatherapy preparations as preservatives. They are natural toners and antiseptics and help the essential oil to dissolve in water and retain its aroma. They are wonderful tonics and rejuvenators for the skin.

Orange flower water/orange leaves – this is great for rejuvenating the skin, also a good relaxer.

Rosewater – this tonic is slightly astringent and has anti-wrinkle properties.

Witch hazel – this is a very good astringent for oily skin, slightly drying.

Yarrow infusion – anti-inflammatory, good for swollen and puffy skin.

Honey

My preference is Manuka honey as it has natural antiseptic and bactericide properties and gives good results in beauty treatments. It originates in New Zealand where it is used by the medical profession to repair, revitalize and soften the skin. It is easily obtained and although it is quite expensive compared to other honeys, it is really worth while.

Clay

White or green clay – this has a cleansing effect on the skin, removing impurities. It is excellent for masks as it boosts circulation and improves the lymphatic flow (lymph is the fluid that surrounds every cell in the body). For normal to oily skins.

Mustard powder

This is a revulsive and makes the skin hot and red – this is the desired effect but don't leave on the skin for longer than ten minutes. Widely available from supermarkets.

Lecithin

Soya protein. You can buy it from health food shops. It is useful for hair preparations (see page 73).

Usage

Infusions

Take a handful of flower petals or bruised herbs or leaves (or one to two tea bags depending on the remedy) and place in a saucepan. Cover with 600ml/1 pint of water and bring to the boil. Take off the heat and let the mixture cool down and 'infuse' for twenty to thirty minutes. Strain and use as advised.

Decoctions

These work on the same principlel as infusions but are made from hard stems, seeds and roots. Use a pestle and mortar to bruise the items before you place in the saucepan, cover with 600ml (1 pint) water and bring to the boil, boiling for five minutes. Infuse for fifteen minutes and strain. Follow individual recipes for quantities.

Tisanes

Tisanes are stronger than teas. Place a handful of leaves, flowers or tea bags (as many as advised) into a teapot and cover with boiling water to clean plant matter. Immediately pour away the water and cover again with 600ml (1 pint) water. Leave for five to seven minutes to infuse then remove the plant matter and drink or use as directed.

Compresses

Compresses can be used hot or cold to reduce swelling and bring down a high temperature. Prepare from a decoction, infusion or tisane. Use a face cloth or piece of gauze and dip into a prepared decoction or tisane. Wring out well. Cover face with cloth and relax for five minutes.

Inhalations

Inhalations cleanse the inside of your body and are extremely useful for congestive ailments, colds and flu, and mucus discharge. They work on the same principle as a facial sauna and you will need a bowl, a towel and your chosen essential oil to add to your boiled hot water. Put the required drops of essential oil in a bowl of hot water and cover your head with the towel, breathing in the fumes for a few minutes.

For a quick fix you can use your hands. Place a drop of essential oil in your warm hands and rub them together vigorously. Cup them over your nose making sure that no air can get in. Inhale deeply for a few moments. This method is good for nausea, panic attacks and stress. Try with rosemary or peppermint.

Poultices

Poultices are very old remedies that soothe irritations, and relieve congestion and pain. Most are made using either linseeds or oatmeal and some gauze cut into two A4 pieces.
If using linseeds – crush three tablespoons lightly in a pestle and mortar, add to a saucepan with enough boiling water to make a paste. Remove from heat. Stir in your essential oil(s).
If using oats – make a porridge from two to three table-spoons of oats and approximately 200ml/7fl oz water. Stir in the essential oils. Then, place one square of gauze on a clean surface. Use a spatula to spread the oats or linseeds onto it, cover with the second gauze square and secure the sides. Place onto the affected area.

Bain-marie

The bain-marie method is often used in making prepara-tions, as it is a good way to melt ingredients slowly.

Stand a bowl in an old saucepan half-filled with boiling water (the water needs to come half-way up the outside of the bowl). Simmer over heat until ingredients have melted.

Essential oils in the bath

Pour the essential oils under running water as directed. Make sure you close the doors and windows so the aromas can't escape. (See also pages 140–43.)

Essential oils in the shower

Put a couple of drops of your selected oils in the shower tray and shower as normal inhaling the fumes. You can also rub the oil on to your body as advised (you could dilute the essential oil in a teaspoon of carrier oil if you have sensitive skin) and the water will release the fumes.

Essential oils in massage

Massage with essential oils is a very effective way of treating ailments. Massage activates nerve endings and stimulates the circulation of blood to the surface of the

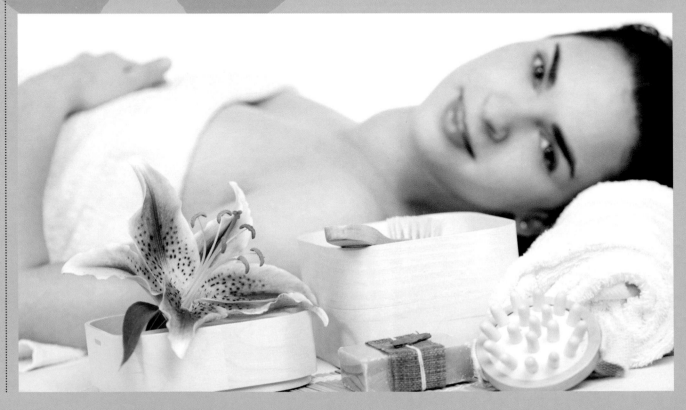

skin, thus easing the entry of oils through the skin. (See pages 146–47) for more information on massage.)

Basic equipment, hygiene and storage

Hygiene

Always wash your hands thoroughly before starting to prepare your remedies – fill a washbasin with warm water and a drop of essential oil of lavender, use this to clean your hands.

Equipment must also be cleaned before use. Add two to three tablespoons cider vinegar to a bowl of boiling water and plunge in your instruments. Keep your equipment in a clean cupboard or bag and use it only for your remedies (don't be tempted to use a wooden spoon from the kitchen for instance!). You should also sterilize all glass bottles and jars for storing remedies in. Wash these in boiling water, then add a couple of drops of tea tree oil and wipe with cotton wool. Give a final rinse again in boiled water.

Storage

Always try to buy dark bottles to store your remedies in to avoid light exposure and damage. Store remedies in a cool, dark place, or in the fridge if directed. Don't use plastic containers as some essential oils will penetrate the plastic.

Useful equipment

Check remedies in advance to make sure you have any equipment you need and make sure everything is clean (see above) before you start. You can buy storage bottles from chemist shops or specialist aromatherapy outlets or you can recycle old medicine bottles and cosmetic jars. Small size measuring glasses can be purchased from cookware shops or from specialist aromatherapy retailers but I have given spoon conversions in the recipes for ease of use. Standard kitchen measuring jugs start from 50ml upwards so these can be used for larger quantities. The following checklist will give you an idea of the sorts of items you will need.

Equipment checklist

Kettle

Tray

Chopping board

Saucepan (old)

China/porcelain bowl (for bain-marie method)

Large bowl for room fragrances and inhalation

Teapot

Tea cup (150ml)

Glasses (small/100ml, medium/150ml, large/250ml)

Measuring jug

Eggcup

Glass containers for dried plant material (rose petals, mint etc.)

Rolling pin to crush seeds etc.

Pestle and mortar

Spatulas, wooden spoons

Cocktail sticks (to act as droppers)

Tongs to pick up dried plants

Glass dropper

Cotton buds

Gauze

Cotton pads

Flannels or old towels

Kitchen rolls and tissues

Coffee filters

Spoons (tea, dessert, table)

Glass bottles, dark, 50ml, 200ml, 1litre, 2 litres

Glass jars and containers, with tops, 10ml, 50ml, 100ml, 200ml

Spray bottle (small), garden spray bottle (large)

Labels (to write date of preparation)

part one

PLANTS & OILS

FOR BEAUTY AND ANTI-AGEING

Angelica archangelica/Archangelica officinalis – Umbelliferae

Angelica

Cultivated in many European countries, Scandinavia, China and northern India, angelica has long been recognized for its medicinal properties.

Benefits

* Stimulant
* Stomachic
* Expectorant
* Tonic for the nervous system
* Blood cleanser
* Elixir for long life
* Restores and repairs the skin
* Relaxes muscles
* Good for memory

Legend has it that during a terrible plague an angel revealed the benefits of angelica to a monk, hence its nickname 'root of the Holy Ghost'. The plant was said to bring luck, protect against illness and greatly extend life – old Provençal folklore tells of a man who lived until 120 all because he chewed the roots of angelica every day (this came with the added bonus of keeping his teeth intact too).

Many old books mention the preventive properties of angelica. John Gerard, herbalist to James I, advised people to chew the stems and to boil the roots, seeds and leaves in order to disinfect their homes and prevent the spread of disease.

Angelica has a ridged, hollow stem and large leaves and is best harvested before it is fully matured. In 1640, the English herbalist John Parkinson pointed out that it should be gathered on a sunny, dry day, thus preserving

Angelica has great rejuvenating and firming properties, and is wonderful for the circulation. It is an excellent natural healer, restoring and repairing.

the medicinal properties. The whole plant – leaves, stems, flowers and seeds – can be used in teas but it must be stored in an airtight, earthenware container.

In Malaysia I was told by a Chinese herbalist that angelica is considered to be particularly good for women and can have great results in helping with post-natal depression, pre-menstrual syndrome (PMS) and the menopause.

I was introduced to the healing properties of angelica by my mentor, Marguerite Maury. She used it in many skin-care preparations as it has great rejuvenating and firming properties, and is wonderful for the circulation. It stimulates skin cells too and is therefore an excellent natural healer, restoring and repairing. You can even use it on stretchmarks!

There are two types of essential oil of angelica – one distilled from the roots and one from the seeds. The seeds contain more essential oil but the oil from the roots is far stronger and more concentrated. I prefer the oil distilled from the seeds, as it is more liquid and therefore easier to use. It is also possible to buy oil that is a combination of the two but check the consistency first. It takes 300kg (660lb) of roots to make just 1kg (2¼lb) of essential oil. It is yellow in colour and quite thick, and mixes well with citrus oils. It has a pungent, earthy smell that takes a while to get used to, but persevere and you will reap the benefits!

Dangers

Essential oil of angelica contains furocoumarines that can cause dermatitis if exposed to sun or ultraviolet light straight after use.

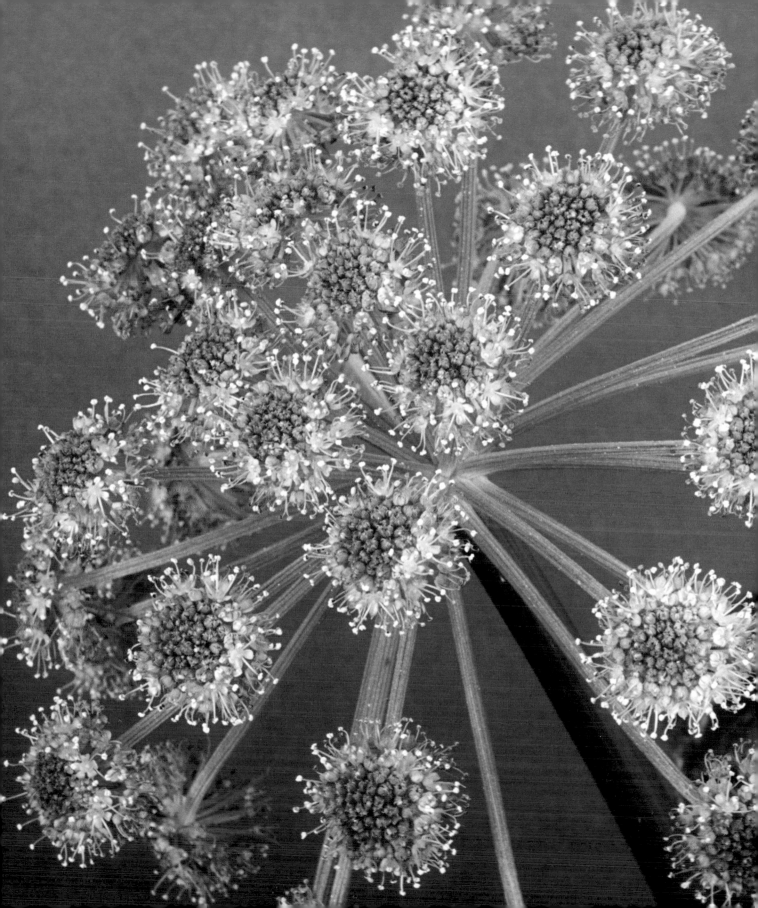

Aniba rosaeodora – Convolvulus scoparius

Bois de rose

The bois de rose tree originates from Africa and South America (Brazil and Equador), where it grows in abundance in the Amazon rainforest.

Benefits

* Rejuvenates and tones skin
* Good for wrinkles and deep expression lines
* Helps with stretchmarks
* Hormonal stimulant
* Helps with nervous disorders
* Used in perfume

Especially good quality bois de rose oil is produced in Guyana. The essential oil is called 'oleo de Pau-Rosa' in Brazil, and its production contributes to huge areas of deforestation in the Amazon, so Brazilian bois de rose should not be purchased.

In the old days bois de rose was used to make expensive furniture as it was easy to carve. The finished piece smelt wonderful and kept insects away.

The gentle aroma of bois de rose is woody and mossy with rose notes. It is a great natural fixative as it has a viscosity and thickness favoured by the perfume industry. The principal constituent is linalool (70–80%), which is often reproduced synthetically. Oils such as lavender, aspic, lemon, thyme and ylang-ylang can be substituted for bois de rose when it is in short supply due to the demands of the perfume industry, and these will all have the same medicinal qualities.

Bois de rose is particularly good for sensitive skins. It can be found in many beauty products to help fight anti-ageing. The people of the Amazon use the essential oil for their skin, to rejuvenate and revitalize.

Dangers

Some oils contain synthetic linalool but still call themselves bois de rose – be wary when buying.

Apium graveolens – Umbelliferae

Celery

The first record of the cultivation of celery was in seventeenth-century France, but it may have been developed in Italy earlier than this.

Benefits

* Anti-ageing
* Combats cellulite
* Tonic for the nervous system
* Strong diuretic
* Blood cleanser
* Aphrodisiac
* Helps coughs
* Helps liver problems

The Greeks called it *selinon* or moon plant as eating celery at full moon was said to act as a tonic and to aid the nervous system. The Romans avoided hangovers by weaving the leaves around their heads and Hippocrates favoured its diuretic properties.

The plant is very pungent in both aroma and flavour. It is extremely diuretic and will help to eliminate toxins. Use in the bath, as a massage oil or as a compress (see page 11).

The essential oil is very pale yellow and fluid. It is distilled from the seeds and has a strong celery smell. Its diuretic properties come from the constituents limonene and selinene, and I have found the essential oil very useful in slimming gels and creams.

Dangers

Because of its strongly diuretic properties, avoid during pregnancy.

Boswellia carteri – Burseraceae
Frankincense

Frankincense is grown in Africa, the Middle East and Oman.

Benefits
* Helps with respiratory problems
* Antiseptic
* Sedative

An aromatic gum resin that comes from a tree of the *Boswellia* family, frankincense has been used for many centuries in religious rituals and is still used today in the form of church incense. Ancient cultures held it in high regard and it was, of course, one of the three gifts given to the baby Jesus.

Frankincense, also known as olibanum, was mentioned by Ancient Greek physician Dioscorides as a treatment for skin disorders, eye problems and pneumonia. Dr Nicolas Lemery (a prominent French doctor and chemist writing in the late seventeenth century) noted that it helped scar tissue to form quickly and, as a result, soldiers were treated with it.

To obtain the essential oil, cuts are made in the tree and a white gum is slowly released. These tear-shaped drops soon dry and fall to the ground where they are collected. Colourless or pale yellow oil is then steam-distilled from the gum. It smells slightly balsamic, lemony with a note of camphor.

Frankincense, also known as olibanum, was mentioned by Ancient Greek physician Dioscorides as a treatment for skin disorders, eye problems and pneumonia.

Calendula officinalis – Compositae
Calendula

The pot marigold, from which calendula oil is obtained, is native to southern Europe.

Benefits
* Helps all skin problems: acne; dermatitis; burns; broken capillaries
* Helps with PMS
* Sudorific (sweat-inducing)
* Tonic
* Emmenagogic (induces menstruation)
* Anti-spasmodic

Calendula has daisy-like flowers that can vary from yellow to orange. The name marigold comes from the Anglo-Saxon *merso-meargealla* or marsh marigold.

Traditionally, if the flowers are cut when the sun is at its highest, the flowers are said to act as a heart tonic and fortifier. Old French texts claim that marigolds can strengthen weak eyes just by looking at them.

The essential oil of calendula is distilled from the flower tops. It has an odd smell that does not appeal to everyone.

Marigolds have been used for centuries to treat skin problems – marigold poultices were used to help heal smallpox scars. Nowadays, calendula is held in high regard in much homoeopathic and holistic medicine.

Cananga odorata – Anonaceae

Ylang-ylang

Ylang-ylang originates from a tree in the Philippines known as the perfume tree. These trees now grow throughout tropical Asia and in Tahiti and were introduced to the island of Réunion in 1884, and from there they were brought to Mauritius and Madagascar.

Benefits

* Soothing
* Aids healing
* Aids anxiety
* Tonic
* Blood cleanser
* Antiseptic for the urinary system, helps with cystitis
* Sexual stimulant, helps with lowered libido
* Helps to top up energy and recharge batteries
* Regulates nervous and emotional tendencies
* Used in perfume

Ylang-ylang is a tree of about 30m (100ft), and looks very similar to the weeping willow. Its flowers are yellowy white and bloom constantly but it is during the rainy season that the tree is particularly loaded with blooms. They have an intoxicating smell that is similar to that of hyacinth and narcissus but with a fresher note.

The fragrant flowers are steam-distilled to produce the essential oil. In order to preserve the aromatic substances, the distillation process begins almost immediately after harvest. Complete extraction can take over twenty-two hours but it is a fractional process as, just like olive oil, you can obtain different qualities – ylang-ylang extra, 1st grade, 2nd grade and so on. I have always insisted on using the best quality for external use. Lesser qualities can be used for baths, showers, candles and in home products.

The principal constituents of ylang-ylang oil are linalool and geraniol. These provide the fresh floral notes reminiscent of hyacinth and narcissus, and make ylang-ylang much sought-after in the perfume industry.

The flowers have been used for their curative properties for centuries. When I was in Malaysia I was told that the locals used to spread the flowers on the beds of newly-weds. They called it Alang-ylang and the scent was meant to mentally prepare the spirit for the act of love – a natural viagra! French phytotherapist Dr Leclerc prescribed it for low libido. Research has also found that ylang-ylang has good results in treating malaria, typhus and other fevers.

Ylang-ylang added to body lotion helps prolong a tan and restores and refreshes the skin.

Marguerite Maury has suggested that, when inhaled, ylang-ylang calms down anger and frustration. Carry a bottle of the essential oil in your bag and, when needed, a few drops on a tissue, inhaled deeply for a few minutes, will be extremely beneficial.

Dangers

Never take ylang-ylang oil internally; it can cause death. Also, beware of an oil called *cananga* that is often sold as ylang-ylang. This is a cheap and inferior quality oil.

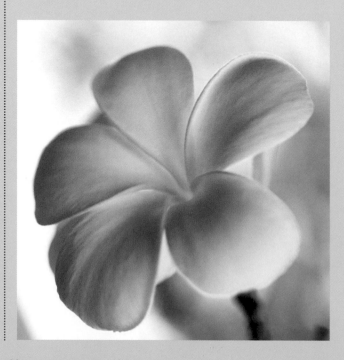

Cedrus atlantica Manetti – Pinaceae

Cedarwood

True cedar, *C. atlantica*, comes from the Atlas Mountains in Morocco – this variety provides the best essential oil for use in therapy.

Benefits

✳ Excellent for healing dermatitis, skin eruptions
✳ Helps dandruff and alopecia
✳ Soothing
✳ Antiseptic
✳ Anti-inflammatory
✳ Aids healing
✳ Respiratory problems
✳ Relaxing
✳ Stimulant

King Solomon was said to have built his temple from cedarwood and it can only be imagined how wonderful it must have been. The wood was used by the Romans to carve out figurines of family members. Kept in the pocket, they would be used in prayer in order to bring health and protection to the person they resembled. Soldiers would take them into battle to protect themselves. Cedarwood was also carved into scented torches for use in the home – the essential oils within the wood helped them to burn, creating a blue glow, and the fragrance provided antiseptic protection against insects and disease. The Ancient Egyptians used cedarwood in embalming and the Sioux Indians burnt it in religious rituals.

The oil is steam-distilled and is yellowish in colour and syrupy in texture. It has a strong smell reminiscent of both pine and honey, with subtle notes of sandalwood.

Cedarwood is particularly good in treating skin eruptions, dermatitis and eczema. It also has a beneficial effect on dandruff and alopecia.

The constituents include terpenic hydrocarbons, some cedrol and sesquiterpenes such as cadinene, which make up its antiseptic and anti-inflammatory properties.

Cedarwood is particularly good in treating skin eruptions, dermatitis and eczema. It also has a beneficial effect on dandruff and alopecia, and in France it is added to specialist shampoos for the latter.

Dangers

The 'cedarwood' oil that originates in the USA comes from junipers *J. flaccida*, *mexicano* and *virginiana*. These are actually all species of juniper and are rich in thujone, found in the constituent cedrol. Thujone is often used to falsify sage oil and is not recommended for external application. Nowadays this variety is only used in soap and perfume. When buying cedarwood essential oil for therapeutic purposes, be sure to source the Moroccan variety.

Chamaemelum nobile; Matricaria chamomilla/recutita – Compositae

Chamomile

Chamomile is cultivated in Morocco, Egypt (a country that is a great producer of organic essential oil) and France (where organic essential oils have flourished for at least the last ten years).

Benefits

* Helps with irregular periods, PMS
* Soothes burns, sunburn
* Helps with skin conditions such as psoriasis, eczema, dermatitis, acne
* Toner
* Eases sensitive skin
* Helps eye infections
* Hair care
* Helps asthma, bronchitis, coughs
* Soothes headaches and migraines
* Helps with digestive problems
* Soothes earache, toothache, neuralgia
* Reduces fever

So many varieties of chamomile exist but the most common is Roman chamomile (*Chamaemelum nobile* or 'the oldest favourites'). Wild or German chamomile (*Matricaria chamomilla* or *recutita*) is very aromatic and has a strange, bitter taste. Both varieties are equally important and widely used in aromatherapy. The scent of chamomile is easy to recognize and you only have to lightly tread on a plant for it to release its fragrance. Many people consider its aroma unpleasant but I find it fruity, sugary and herby, and it instantly makes me feel comforted and reassured.

Chamaemelum is derived from the Greek for 'apples on the ground' as the plant is low-lying and the flowers have an apple scent. For the same reason, in Spain it is called *manzanilla* or 'little apple'. *Matricaria* comes from the Latin word *matrix* or 'womb', which may offer a clue to its use, as it is helpful for all manner of menstrual problems. The Ancient Greeks used it to treat young girls with menstrual difficulties and their name for the plant was *parthenos* or 'girl'.

In northern France the yellow chamomile was thought of as a sacred plant. Similar in shape to the yellow disc of the sun, it was offered to the sun god Baldur in the hope that he would grant good fortune and success in cultivating crops in return. The Ancient Egyptians also considered it sacred and dedicated it to Râ, the god of the sun. They understood its therapeutic value and placed it in tombs next to mummies in case they might need it in their next life. In order to get a good night's sleep, the Elizabethans in Britain would smoke it. Chamomile is particularly noted for its ability to bring down fever, and in case of this the Ancient Greek physician Dioscorides recommended crushing the flowers to a powder and taking it with water.

In 1697 Dr Nicolas Lemery called it the universal remedy for women, while in 1876 Dr Cazin wrote in his *Traité Pratique et Raisonné des Plantes Medicinales* that chamomile was the best treatment for rheumatic and digestive conditions, and gout.

The main constituent of the essential oil of chamomile is azulene, which is an anti-inflammatory and promotes quick healing of the skin. A higher proportion of azulene is found in the plants at dawn and dusk, so they tend to be picked at these times. The oil is slightly bluish in colour; if it's brownish-yellow it has passed its sell-by date!

Most people have heard of chamomile tea but there are many other ways to utilize its many wonderful properties. Culpeper, in his Herbal, advised its use as a tonic or to calm a hysterical or nervous disposition (presumably because it soothes and sedates). When I was a little girl it was used for bruises, eye infections, stomach aches, growing pains, cuts and burns, and put in baby lotions, bath treatments, hair rinses… It is especially good for many skin problems, such as acne and eczema. A used chamomile teabag will help reduce puffiness around the eyes. It is a common ingredient in hair products for fair hair.

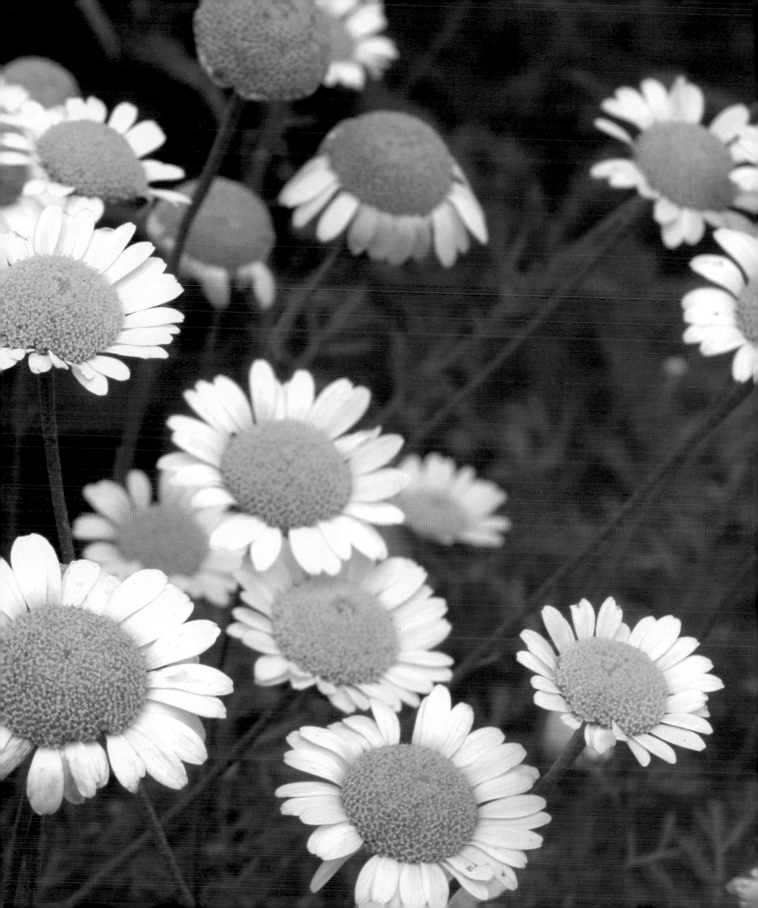

Cinnamomum zeylanicum/Cinnamomum cassia – Lauraceae

Cinnamon

This tree is purported to have originated in China or Burma but is now cultivated in many tropical countries.

Benefits

* Anti-bactericide
* Immunostimulant
* Disinfectant
* Anti-viral
* Pick-me-up
* Treats mouth ulcers
* Helps with flu and respiratory problems

Cinnamon comes from the bark of trees belonging to the laurel family. The evergreen tree exudes a spicy aroma and can grow to a height of 18m (60ft). It has shiny leaves and yellow flowers that grow in clusters.

Cinnamon was mentioned in Pen T'sao, 'the Divine Healer', Emperor Shen Nung's treatise in 2700 BC. At the time, the Chinese prescribed it for everything (as a tranquillizer, tonic and for depression). It was used in Ancient Egypt in embalming and for keeping epidemics at bay.

When the tree is approximately six years old, the bark is delicately removed in lengthy strips before being left to dry in the sun. This is done every second year and the tree can carry on producing the bark for over 200 years.

The bark, leaves and twigs are all used for the distillation of the essential oil. The main constituent is cinnamic aldehyde (60–65%), which is a warming and strong antiseptic. Methylamine ketone gives the oil its aroma.

Nowadays, of course, cinnamon is the mainstay of many baking recipes, curries, drinks etc. It gives a spicy note to perfumes and eau de toilettes, and is a favourite ingredient of men's cosmetics and soap.

Dangers

Cinnamon essential oil can be toxic and is not advised for use on people with sensitive skin. It must always be well diluted with other essential oils and carrier oils. Never add to a hot bath.

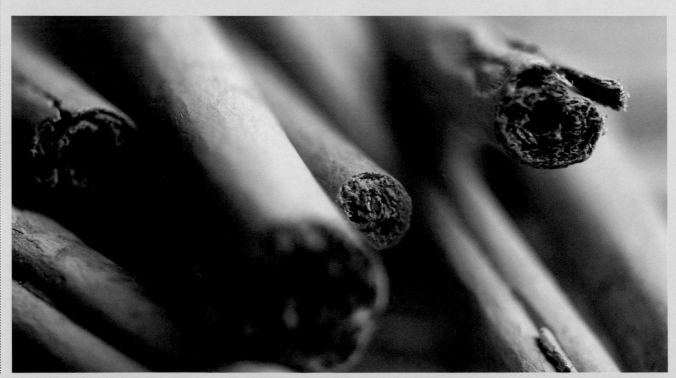

Citrus aurantifolia/latifolia – Rutaceae

Lime/Limette

Most lime essential oil comes from Mexico, Florida, Trinidad, Haiti and Jamaica. Limette is the name used in the fragrance industry.

Benefits
* Antiseptic
* Natural antibiotic
* Rejuvenates and softens skin

The essential oil is extracted from the zest of *C. aurantifolia* and *latifolia*. The oil is easier to obtain from the former variety; the latter is only available to a very select clientele. Over 900 tonnes of the essential oil is extracted every year.

The essential oil is golden and somewhat reminiscent of bergamot but the aroma is more subtle and intense. The principal constituents are citral and linalyl acetate, which are strong antiseptics and bactericides.

Lime essential oil is used to aromatize drinks and also used in houschold products. It is refreshing and good to use as a vaporizer because of its antiseptic properties. It mixes well with many other essential oils.

If you cannot get hold of the essential oil you can use fresh limes. Peel, chop and boil the skins of two to three large, unwaxed and thoroughly washed limes in 600ml (1 pint) of water. Boil gently for fifteen minutes and then reduce the heat for a further five minutes. When cool you can add this to bath water for a rejuvenating, refreshing and skin-softening bath.

The essential oil is golden and somewhat reminiscent of bergamot but the aroma is more subtle and intense.

Citrus aurantium bergamia – Rutaceae

Bergamot

The bergamot tree is said to have originated in India but nowadays its main habitat is southern Italy, the Ivory Coast and the Republic of Guinea. Christopher Columbus reportedly exported the tree from the Canary Islands to the New World.

Benefits
* Anti-ageing
* Anti-spasmodic
* Antiseptic
* Tonic
* Digestive
* Helps with loss of appetite
* Eases anxiety

The bergamot tree is smaller in size than the other citrus varieties. It has smallish, pear-shaped fruits and has been mentioned in herbals since the sixteenth century.

The essential oil is a lovely emerald colour and is extracted from the fruits. The main constituent is linalyl acetate but it also contains the furocoumarines, bergamontine and bergaptene. These two constituents increase the production of melanin in the skin and the oil should therefore never be used before exposure to the sun. Do not use it in the bath, for example, before going out in the sun, and never use it if you have large moles. Used wrongly, the essential oil can accelerate skin problems such as dermatitis, pigmentation spots and lesions, and because of this, I prefer not to use it much in skin care. It is, however, a great tonic and I use the fruit for many digestive ailments and for anxiety.

Bergamot is used as a flavouring in Earl Grey tea and as a scent in many cosmetics. The best way to reap its benefits is to add a few drops of the essential oil to bowls of hot water and place them around your home. It has a tonic effect on the nervous system, soothing one's mind after a late night, and aiding recuperation after stress and fatigue.

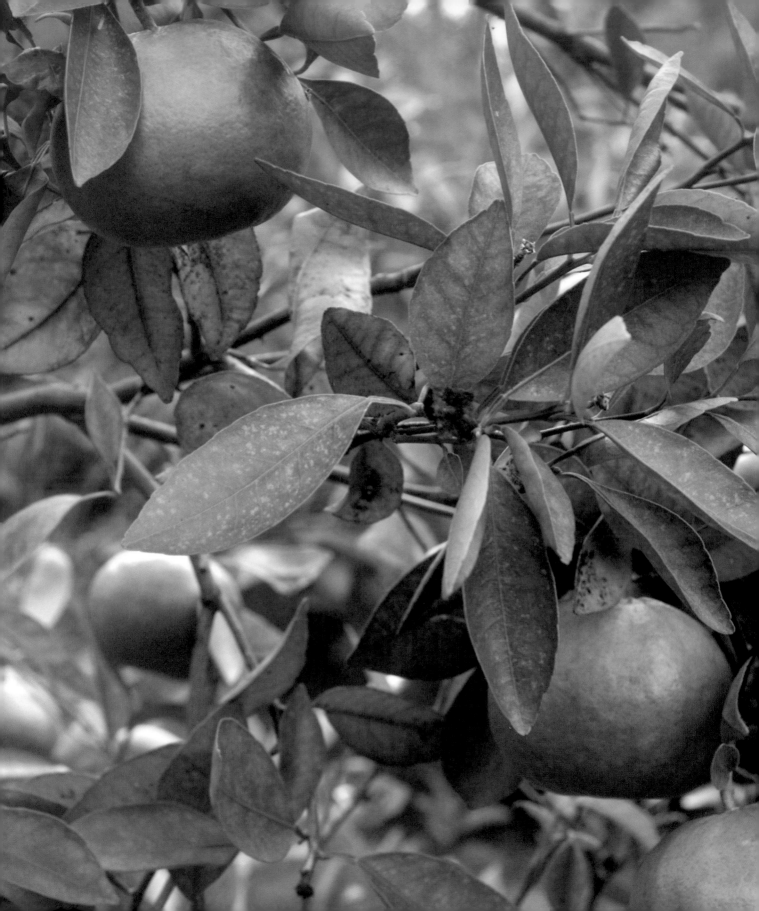

Citrus aurantium sinensis – Rutaceae

Orange

The origin of the orange is in China but oranges now grow in most countries with hot climates. The principal producers are Spain, Italy, North Africa and Egypt.

Benefits

✻ Anti-ageing
✻ Rejuvenates skin and combats wrinkles
✻ Helps with couperose (prominent veins)
✻ Soothes nervous tension and anxiety
✻ Aids fatigue
✻ Sedative
✻ Helps with muscle cramps
✻ Treats alopecia
✻ Good for tooth decay, bad breath, gingivitis, gum sensitivity

The orange tree is remarkable because every part is utilized for essential oil. The leaves produce petit grain – one of the most important essential oils in aromatherapy (see page 28). The beautifully scented flowers produce essential oil of neroli (see page 28) and the skins of the oranges themselves make essential oil of orange. Orange wood itself was once carved into handles for tools.

For each thousand oranges you may be able to produce 500g (1 lb) essential oil, but this depends on the climate, seasons and the weather (an important factor in the maturing of the fruits). Over 90% of the oil is made up of limonene, a strong antiseptic. Of the other components, citral gives the essential oil its bactericide properties, while geraniol and linalool are known for their rejuvenating properties.

When buying actual oranges, always buy them unwaxed and make sure that they haven't been sprayed with ethylene. The skins must be supple. Always wash them in warm water before juicing them.

The medicinal properties of oranges were discovered towards the end of the sixteenth century. Oranges soon found their place among Christmas and New Year festivities and became a favoured gift – I remember my grandparents talking about receiving oranges as a special Christmas gift. The French Pharmocopae advised that the skin be dried then stewed and then given to patients in the form of a drink to treat night fever. Orange skin was also used to treat constipation and classified as a good diuretic.

In 1690, Dr Lazar prescribed orange skin for vertigo, heart palpitations, asthma, travel sickness and post-labour pain.

I have successfully used essential oil of orange to treat vein problems, couperose, thread veins, aiding micro-circulation and skin congestion. It is also wonderful for wrinkles.

In France you can buy orange seeds, crush them and drink in tisanes (see page 11) – a great way to detoxify your body. The fruit has so many rejuvenating properties because of its bioflavanoid complex (this helps fortify the capillaries, veins and vascular system). Vitamins B and C are also good for keeping the skin healthy and oranges are full of minerals like calcium, magnesium, phosphorous, potassium, copper and sulphur – all good for general health. The juice helps stimulate the immune system, thus protecting against colds and flu. In France there is a proverb about oranges; 'gold in the morning to drink, silver at lunch and lead in the evening', in other words, the earlier in the day you drink orange juice, the better it is for you.

Dangers

Make sure you buy a fresh supply of orange oil – the colour must be a nice pale orange and have a pleasant smell. If the oil is brown in colour and has a fishy smell, dispose of it.

See also Neroli *and* Petit Grain *overleaf, which are both from the orange tree too.*

Citrus aurantium bigaradia – Rutaceae

Neroli

Neroli is distilled in the south of France, Italy, Spain, Sicily and North Africa.

Benefits

❋ Helps with skin eruptions, acne, eczema
❋ Improves micro-circulation
❋ Aids nervous tension
❋ Helps with PMS and menopausal problems
❋ Eases insomnia
❋ Helps with hangovers
❋ Used in perfume

Neroli is a wonderful essence with a sumptuous, sweet, sensuous and heady aroma. The essential oil is obtained from the fresh flowers of the orange tree. It takes more than a tonne of flowers to produce a kilo (2¼lb) of essential oil and, as a result, the oil is one of the most expensive. The *bigaradia* variety is the most favoured because it has a rich aroma. The essence is known as 'Neroli Bigaradia' with the other variety available being *Citrus aurantium*, 'Neroli Portugal'.

Neroli oil is thought to have been named after Anna Maria de la Tremoille, princess of Neroli, a small town near Rome. It was said to be Napoleon's favourite fragrance, reminding him of his beloved Corsica. When he became emperor, he was given a perfume and soap containing neroli essential oil. The soap was later made available for everyone to buy.

Essential oil of neroli is yellow at first but when exposed to air, it becomes reddish brown. One of its constituents is jasmone, which gives neroli its sweet scent, while nerol gives the oil its sedative properties.

Neroli is revered in aromatherapy for its calming properties. It is wonderful as a constituent of massage oils, bath essences and as a natural perfume. When I make up my own perfumes I always give neroli a '*place d'honneur*'.

My family added orange flowers to crème caramel, cakes and teas. They were given to me when I was little to calm me down and aid sleep. They are also great for colicky babies – just add a tablespoon of an infusion (see page 11) to their milk.

Orange-flower water, or *aquaflorum naphae*, as it was known to the Ancients, is highly valued. Its rejuvenating properties accelerate the production of skin cells, it is a wonderful calmer and fortifier for the nervous system, and can be used as a gentle antiseptic for acne (especially for those with sensitive skin). It is used regularly as much in cosmetics as it is in cooking in many countries.

Citrus aurantium bigaradia – Rutaceae

Petit Grain

Petit grain was one of the first essential oils to be produced in Grasse in France (a world centre of the perfume industry), but nowadays it comes from South America. Most of this oil is used in perfumery (often as a base for eau de toilette and flower water), cosmetics and for flavouring in the food industry.

Benefits

❋ Helps with facial/jaw stiffness
❋ Smoothing, rejuvenating
❋ Gentle antiseptic – good for pimples/spots
❋ Helps insomnia, fear
❋ Used in perfume

The leaves of the orange tree are distilled to produce petit grain. The tree needs strong cutting back every two years before the leaves are distilled together with the small green fruits.

The scent of petit grain is fresher than that of orange. It is good for all the relaxing treatments and has similar properties to orange but is more subtle and less definite. Neat oil applied with a cottonbud is wonderful for spots and pimples. Petit grain leaves can be used in decoctions (see page 11) for their digestive and calming properties.

Citrus paradisi – Rutaceae

Grapefruit

Grapefruit originates in California and comes from the same family as mandarin, lemon and orange.

Benefits

* Improves cellulite, stretchmarks
* Helps acne, greasy skin
* Eases fatigue
* Helps with muscular cramps
* Treats hair loss
* Stimulant
* Detoxifier
* Aids lymphatic drainage

Grapefruit seeds are now used as natural preservatives, instead of parabens, in many skin-care products. The essential oil is very useful for treating cellulite and fluid retention, stretchmarks and acne. Grapefruit makes a wonderful perfume and can be used in the bath or diffused in a room.

The essential oil is obtained from the zest and it contains at least 60% limonene, citral and citronellol.

Dangers

It is always best to buy organic because sometimes traces of pesticides can be found in the oil. This is particularly true of citrus oils in general.

Grapefruit seeds are now used as natural preservatives, instead of parabens, in many skin-care products.

Citrus reticulata, C. nobilis, C. madurensis – Rutaceae

Mandarin

The mandarin tree originates from the southern Chinese province of Yunnan. It is now cultivated in Japan, Burma and India, and production is starting in Tahiti and the USA.

Benefits

* Tonic
* Stomachic
* Slightly hypnotic
* Bactericide
* Treats nervous disorders such as insomnia

The mandarin tree is approximately 5–8m (16–26ft) in height. Numerous hybrids have been cultivated since the old times – tangerine and clementine are just two of them. Mandarin is different from the other varieties because of its little leaves and small orange or green fruits. The delicate fruits with the soft, pulpy centres and agreeable aroma make it one of the most appreciated plants.

The name comes from Mandarin Chinese; the fruits were often given by them as a gift. It is also purported that they wore clothes with buttons shaped like the fruit.

The skin of the mandarin contains a wonderful essential oil that is extracted by cold expression in the same way as the other citrus fruits. It is a golden colour with a light blue/violet iridescence. Its smell is somewhere between lemon and orange but more agreeable to the nose with a slightly sweeter note.

Citrus limon – Rutaceae

Lemon

Lemon originated from China, Japan, Southeast Asia and India. The Arabs later introduced it to Europe from the forests of north India. Nowadays you can find lemon trees growing on the west coast of America and throughout the Mediterranean.

Benefits

* ✳ Tonic for the nervous system
* ✳ Reduces stress
* ✳ Helps with depression
* ✳ Curative properties
* ✳ Bactericide
* ✳ Protects against infections
* ✳ Antiseptic
* ✳ Immunostimulant
* ✳ Fungicide
* ✳ Aids concentration
* ✳ Rejuvenating

The trees can produce over 1500 fruits a year and the flowers have the most exquisite and unique aroma. The floral notes of bergamotine and limettine are literally out of this world. Lemon trees surrounded the house in which I lived in Trinidad in the Caribbean and it was always such a pleasure to open the windows and breathe in the wonderful scent. It was only later when studying that I found out how lemon helps to alleviate tiredness and stress – no wonder I felt so good near the trees!

The exotic aroma of lemon was recorded in ancient scripts as far back as 10 BC and it was referred to in ancient Arab culture as the medicinal apple. The Ancient Egyptians and later the Greeks used them in religious ceremonies and hieroglyphics now reveal that they were revered for their power to protect against spells. In the French Royal Court during the reign of Louis XIV, women used half a lemon in place of lipstick – they would bite on it intermittently and the acid would keep their lips plump and rosy. Visitors to the court were also offered lemons as a welcoming gift. People also used to place lemon peel inside their clothes to keep insects off the fabric. But perhaps most famously in history, the British gave them to their sailors along with limes to combat scurvy.

Lemon has a place in rejuvenation and health today, and is used in many beauty products. Its restoring and healing properties mean it is a wonderful ingredient in a toner or face mask.

The citral content also makes it a marvellous antiseptic and bactericide – great for cleaning hands and under nails! Lemon is the most common distilled essential oil after orange and can also be found in perfumes, household products and cakes.

Lemon is very useful in times of stress; as a juice it is a wonderful detoxifier first thing in the morning, it helps keep you youthful and is excellent for rheumatic conditions as it helps keep the body supple. If I have a gastric problem I take lemon – the enzymes in it help break down food, which can be really helpful.

The essential oil is a polyvalent (cure-all) and a lot of research has been done to prove its bactericidal and antiseptic effect. The oil is pale yellow with a fresh smell. The principal constituents are limonene and citral, which makes it one of the top antiseptics.

Dangers

In general, citrus oils don't keep for too long – the aroma becomes disagreeable and fishy. Make sure that you check the date and consistency (it shouldn't be cloudy) when you buy it.

Lemon has a place in rejuvenation and health today, and is used in many beauty products. Its restoring and healing properties mean it is a wonderful ingredient in a toner or face mask.

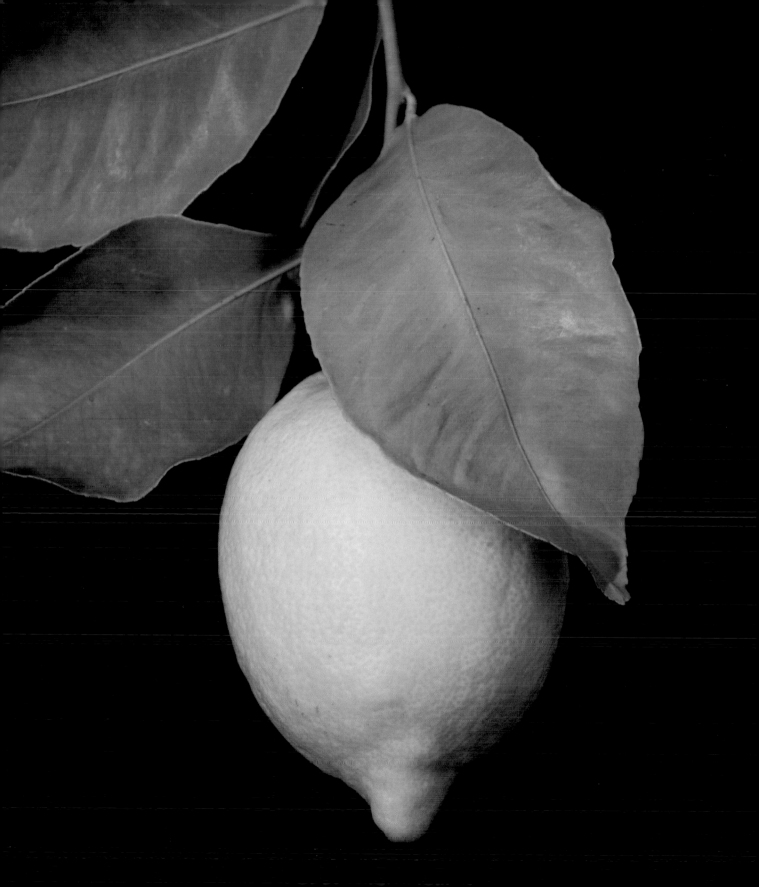

Commiphora myrrha – Burseraceae

Myrrh

Myrrh comes from a tree that originates in Africa (Somalia, Libya and Ethiopia) and Yemen.

Benefits

* Helps with pulmonary problems
* Expectorant
* Gives texture, shine and hold to hair
* Natural UV filter of 3–5 SPF
* Astringent
* Anti-inflammatory
* Healing and rejuvenating: acne, dermatitis and scars
* Antiseptic: good for throat and gum problems
* Sedative: calms emotions
* Stimulant
* Natural fixative in perfumes

The gum of the myrrh tree is distilled to produce the essential oil, which is a dark orangey-yellow. It is well known in the cosmetic and perfume industries for its slightly musky, camphory, spicy hot smell. The principal constituents are acids, phenols and resins, which make the oil balsamic and, in turn, good for the lungs and chest. The oil is quite expensive and can be often falsified – if the colour is a reddish-brown it will probably be adulterated with a solvent.

Myrrh has been mentioned in the Bible and many other religious treatises such as the Koran and the Egyptian Papyris. It was well known to the Ancients and was one of the ingredients used in religious ceremonies and fumigations by the Egyptians.

Many remedies like 'l'elixir de Carus', 'baume de Fioraventi' and 'baume de commandeur' included myrrh. They helped ease pain, and heal cuts, wounds and burns. Dr Nicolas Lemery, in his *Traite des Drogues Simples*, advised its use in facilitating labour while it has also been recorded as being excellent in the treatment of skin diseases and as a good antiseptic for rotten teeth.

Coriandrum sativum – Umbelliferae

Coriander

Coriander is found in southern Europe, Russia, North Africa and South America.

Benefits

* Helps with facial stiffness and cramps
* Soothes toothache
* Helps with flu, fevers
* Eases rheumatic conditions

Coriander can grow up to 30–60cm (1–2ft). It has bright green leaves with whitish, mauvish flowers.

The name coriander comes from the Greek *koris*, meaning bug, as there is apparently a connection between the smell of the leaves and that of bed bugs. I think the smell is very aromatic and I associate it with southern cooked dishes and some digestive French liqueurs.

The essential oil is transparent in colour and it takes approx 100kg (220lb) of the plant to produce 1kg (2¼lb) of essential oil.

I have found it helpful in the treatment of neuralgia due to shingles, facial cramps and toothache. Marguerite Maury gave it to patients suffering from rheumatic complaints and fever. In the past it was used in obstetrics – doctors would place a few of the seeds on a woman's thigh during labour; this was said to quicken birth and lessen pain.

Dangers

When using the oil, great care must be taken as it can be very dangerous if used in large quantities. It must never be taken internally.

Cypress

Cupressus sempervirens – Cupressaceae

Around twenty species of conifer form the genus *Cupressus*. This majestic evergreen originated in Mediterranean Europe but can now be found in other temperate European countries and North America.

Benefits

* Helps with thread veins, varicose veins
* Good for menstrual cycle problems
* Eases oedema, bruising
* Helps with fatigue
* Treats circulatory problems (chilblains/frostbite)
* Reduces heavy sweating
* Antiseptic
* Anti-infection

In Ancient times, forests of cypress were found all over Crete. The Greeks dedicated cypress to the god of the underworld, Pluto. As a result, it became a symbol of peace and tranquillity and can often be found in cemeteries. The Ancient Egyptians recorded its medicinal properties and used the wood to make sarcophagi.

Cypress is extremely efficient in treating bruising, respiratory problems and bleeding, and was recommended by both Hippocrates and Dioscorides in Ancient Greek times. Phytotherapist Dr Leclerc gave it to his patients to stem internal bleeding. In Provence in France the tree is used to protect crops from strong winds.

The essential oil has a yellowish tone and a very balsamic, woody aroma. It is produced from the cones and needles and contains the terpines b-pinene and terpinol. These make up at least 65% of the oil and help blood circulation.

Lemongrass

Cymbopogon citratus and *flexuosus* – *Gramineae*

Originating in Asia, lemongrass is now also found in India, Central America, Madagascar and Brazil.

Benefits

* Skin firming action
* Helps re-balance the sebum secretions
* Prevents against open pores
* Helps with muscular fatigue
* Eases nervous tension
* Helps headaches, migraines
* Decongestant
* Antiseptic, anti-inflammatory
* Rejuvenating

Essential oil of lemongrass comes from *C. citratus* while *C. flexuosus* produces the essential oil *verveine des Indes* (Indian verbena). Because of their similar constituents, lemongrass and verveine are often confused.

The grass can reach up to 30–50cm (12–20 inches) in height and needs to be planted six months before it is harvested, with the fresh leaves being cut again to obtain a better yield.

The high citral content of lemongrass (70–85%) means the oil is a wonderful antiseptic, anti-inflammatory and has strong anti-ageing properties. Other constituents, geraniol and nerol, help combat stress and fatigue. The colour of the oil varies from brown to reddish dark brown.

In Ayurvedic medicine, lemongrass is often prescribed for illnesses and viral infections. During my time in Mysore in India, I visited a hospital for a lecture and found that it is often used to disinfect the common areas. It has a lovely pungent aroma of lemon.

Dangers

Essential oil of lemongrass should never be used neat on the skin. The high amounts of citral need to be diluted in a carrier oil or water.

Cymbogopon martini – Gramineae

Palmarosa

Palmarosa originally came from Central and North India and is now grown in Africa, Java, Madagascar and Nepal.

Benefits

* Anti-ageing
* Helps with wrinkles
* Has a firming action when used in the bath
* Rebalances skin secretions
* Aids the healing of boils
* Helps acne, couperose (prominent veins)
* Calming, refreshing action on the skin
* Soothes burns
* Helps urinary infections
* Anti-viral
* Anti-allergenic
* Eases anxiety and fatigue
* Helps promote good digestion

Palmarosa comes from a family of tropical grasses rich in aromatic oils and is closely related to lemongrass and citronella. The grass is slender and has beautiful white flowers that turn from whitish-blue to red in maturity.

The leaves and flowers of both young and mature plants can be used for essential oil – the young plants produce light oil, while the older ones produce oil with a heavy aroma. The oil is also known as the Indian herb, Indian geranium or Turkish geranium oil. (Distilled in Turkey since the eighteenth century, it has been used to simulate or adulterate the very expensive Turkish rose oil.)

Geraniol is the main constituent (between 75-95%), with phenol giving the oil its wonderful anti-bacterial properties – as a result, the oil is a great anti-ageing agent, firming and rejuvenating the skin. It is highly effective for skin conditions such as acne, healing old acne scars and for skin that has become leathery through over exposure to the sun. It is a useful treatment for boils – apply the oil neat to the boil (using a cotton bud) morning and night.

Palmarosa is also used to combat illness. In India, the plant was taken internally as a remedy against fever and infection, relieving the symptoms of flu and a high temperature. It is also good for aiding the healing of cuts and wounds. You can use it in place of lavender when your skin has been burnt, either by the sun or by fire. It has a good refreshing feel on the skin and will help to mask pain. Used in curries and meat dishes it also helps to kill any bacteria and helps the digestion of fats.

Palmarosa has many usages in traditional Ayurvedic medicine, for raising of one's spirit and for coping with the ups and downs that often accompany a woman's menstrual cycle or which occur after giving birth. To stabilize emotions, frequent inhalation of the essential oil is recommended as it can have numerous benefits and help to overcome depression. This rich essential oil is also considered a mental stimulant.

I love its rosy scent, which is gentle and penetrating at the same time. In India, I was told that the Buddha, too, loved its aroma. It is also greatly revered in Tibet and is used regularly there in medicine.

Dangers

The oil can be easily falsified with cheaper oils such as coco oil and gurgum. In the past, the essential oil of palmarosa was itself used to falsify more expensive oils such as rose. It is therefore important to obtain the right essential oil for therapy.

In India, the plant was taken internally as a remedy against fever and infection, relieving the symptoms of flu and a high temperature.

Daucus carota – Umbelliferae

Carrot

Carrots originated in Afghanistan but the Ancient Greeks and Romans also enjoyed them. Nowadays many different varieties exist – my local market in Nice in France used to stock white, deep purple and red ones!

Benefits

* Anti-ageing: helps with wrinkles
* Brings colour to pale complexions
* Helps with thread veins
* Good for dermatitis, acne
* Tonic
* Soothes sunburn
* Blood cleanser
* Helps with gum and mouth problems

The familiar orange carrot *D. carota spp. sativus* was developed by the Dutch in the seventeenth century. The plant has feathery leaves and an acrid aroma.

In sixteenth-century France, carrots were prescribed as a blood cleanser, for liver and skin disorders, and many digestive, respiratory, allergic and nervous disorders.

Carrots are very nutritious and have a wonderful action on the digestive system. They are particularly favoured for their vitamin A content and are very good for eye problems such as blurred vision and tired eyes. (It is even purported that carrots were given to pilots during the Second World War to help improve their night vision.)

The vegetable is a great ally in the war against viruses. Vitamins A, C, D, E, K and B complex all help boost the immune system. The fresh juice helps coughs and is

Carrot is a great essential oil for rejuvenating the skin, especially for those with skin disorders such as psoriasis, dermatitis, acne and sensitive skin, thread veins, loss of tone. It is excellent for regaining firmness and elasticity.

the perfect tonic when you feel rundown. It also helps gum problems, mouth irritations and ulcers, and abscesses.

The essential oil is extracted from the seeds. For the last few decades, many perfumeries have utilized its spicy, peppery note. The smell is not to everyone's liking though, so it's good to mix it with another essential oil that has similar properties (such as galbanum, rose, bois de rose).

The principal constituents of carrot are limonene, terpineol, pinene, cineol and b-carotene, which has good rejuvenating properties. Thus carrot is a great essential oil for rejuvenating the skin, especially for those with skin disorders such as psoriasis, dermatitis, acne and sensitive skin, thread veins, loss of tone. It is excellent for regaining firmness and elasticity.

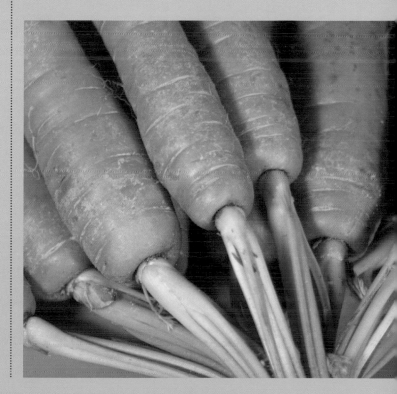

Elettaria cardamomum – Zingiberaceae

Cardamom

Cardamom is a herbaceous perennial that is native to India and Sri Lanka.

Benefits

✳ Natural diuretic: helps with cellulite; slimming; reduces facial puffiness
✳ Helps with PMS and menopausal problems
✳ Good for flatulence, digestion
✳ Warming
✳ Helps with halitosis
✳ Stimulant of the nervous system
✳ Reduces stress and tension
✳ Antiseptic: air freshener; disinfectant

There are many botanical varieties of cardamom but *Elettaria* and *Amomum* are the most common. I came across the *Elettaria* variety when I was living in Mysore, India. It is a herbaceous plant, almost like a small tree, and can grow to approximately 3m (10ft). The leaves are linear and the flowers a magnificent yellow. It has sturdy creeping roots, which indicate its close relationship with ginger. From the base of the plant grow the seedpods that have to be harvested just before ripening. They are brownish in colour and have a peppery, camphory, gingery smell, which I find so agreeable.

The name 'cardamom' is thought to have come from the Arab '*hehmama*', a word derived from the Sanskrit for 'hot and peppery'. The Arabs favoured its diuretic properties. It was used regularly by the Ancient Egyptians and soon found its place in their religious ceremonies and as an integral part of their perfumes. Hippocrates, the Greek physician regarded as the Father of Medicine, praised its aroma and usage in medicine and culinary recipes. Numerous poets have described it as an exquisite aromatic plant.

In Chinese medicine cardamom has numerous medicinal properties but the most important is its action on intestinal problems such as flatulence and constipation. More recently, phytotherapist Dr Leclerc valued it for its carminative (wind expelling), stomachic properties and also as a balm for the nervous system.

I have found it useful for the treatment of stress-related symptoms – lack of sleep, overwork and all the stomach problems related to nervous tension. The aromatic seeds are also great for halitosis and bad breath.

In Oman in the 1970s the locals added cardamom to coffee to accentuate its digestive properties and to add a subtle flavour.

With its strong diuretic properties, it is good for fighting cellulite. In skin care it reduces puffiness and swelling around the face. It brings warmth when added to other essential oils, has wonderful anti-viral and antiseptic properties and can be used to help disinfect the air. Added to perfume it brings a special gingery note.

The essential oil, distilled from the seeds, is a bright yellow colour and very aromatic. Its main constituents are terpineol and cineol, which are both good antioxidants. The small traces of zingiberene give the oil its special aroma. This, however, can vary depending on where the seeds have been distilled.

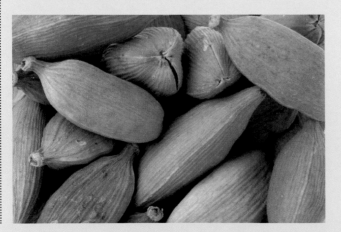

Cardamom was used regularly by the Ancient Egyptians and soon found its place in their religious ceremonies and as an integral part of their perfumes.

Eucalyptus spp. – Myrtaceae

Eucalyptus

The eucalyptus tree originated in Tasmania and was first catalogued by a French explorer in 1792. It was later introduced to the Mediterranean countries and North Africa.

Benefits

* Antiseptic
* Helps respiratory problems such as bronchitis, catarrh, coughing
* Good for urinary infections
* Anti-inflammatory
* Astringent
* Treats rheumatic conditions
* Stimulant of the nervous system, counters fatigue
* Helps with depression
* Treats neuralgia
* Good for spots and pimples

There are approximately 600 species of eucalyptus, or gum trees as they are more commonly known. From these 600 species, only about 15 really have therapeutic properties and, of these, it is the *E. globulus* variety (the Tasmanian blue gum) that is the most esteemed in medicine.

The essential oil is clear and yellow, and transparent and fluid. It has a fresh, balsamic smell. The oil was first distilled in Australia in 1854 and was mentioned by the English surgeon John White who praised its antiseptic properties.

Its principal use is for the respiratory system, treating viral infections such as colds and flu, catarrh, hay fever, and infections of the urinary system such as cystitis. Its antiseptic properties mean it is good in the treatment of spots and pimples.

The trees also help combat malaria in countries with a high risk of the disease. The trees have a great capacity to absorb stagnant water, ridding mosquitoes of their breeding habitats.

Eugenia caryophyllata – Myrtaceae

Clove

Cloves come from a beautiful evergreen tree originating in Mauritius. It has now been introduced to most tropical countries including Madagascar, Tanzania and the Caribbean islands.

Benefits

* Helps with general fatigue
* Good for gum and tooth infections
* Antiseptic and anti-viral
* Stimulates digestion and restores appetite
* Helps rheumatic pains

The clove tree can grow to 10m (30ft) but for cultivation they are kept to a smaller height. The shiny green leaves have visible dots underneath containing aromatic substances that are released when the leaf is bruised. If left to bloom, the tree has lovely crimson flowers that appear at the end of the rainy season. The cloves are these unopened flower buds that are picked by hand before they bloom. They are then left to dry in the sun and soon become the dark brown colour we are familiar with.

When fully matured, each tree can produce over 2kg (4lb) of buds, which represents only 150ml (5fl oz) of essential oil – a lot of work for such a small quantity!

Clove trees used to grow so abundantly on the island of Penang that many believed the strong antiseptic properties of the cloves explained the lack of epidemics on the island. With the destruction of the forests, epidemics came to Penang. Thankfully, the trees are being re-planted.

It is a very useful antiseptic and can be used for the sterilization of surgical instruments and to clean kitchen worktops. In fact pomanders with cloves originated in the Renaissance to keep epidemics and plague at bay.

Dangers

Clove oil should never be used undiluted, neat on the skin or added to a bath unless it is part of a formulation mixed with other essential oils.

Ferula galbaniflua – Umbelliferae

Galbanum

Galbanum grows in southern Europe, North Africa and western Asia, and is thought to have originated in Iran.

Benefits

* Helps wrinkles, crow's-feet, stretchmarks
* Helps nail problems
* Encourages scar tissue to form
* Useful in the treatment of skin problems
* Gives dull hair shine

Galbanum is a gum resin that comes from some *Ferula* species, a perennial plant from the fennel family, with a smooth stem and shiny leaflets. To obtain the resin, the bark and roots are cut to release the sap. The droplets, the size of small nuts, then harden before being picked off for distillation. The resin can be viscous or dry depending on the species of *Ferula* it comes from.

Galbanum has been around since the time of the Ancient Egyptians and Hebrews. Old scriptures mention it by name and it was often used in religious ceremonies. Ancient writers such as Dioscorides and Pliny mentioned its value as a sedative of pain, diuretic and anti-spasmodic. It has also been used to calm night-time hot flushes during the menopause.

Galbanum has a wonderful rejuvenating effect on skin disorders and can help lessen crow's-feet, wrinkles and deep lines. I have also found it helpful in the treatment of stretchmarks, scars, nail problems, dull hair, scalp problems and as a fixative in perfume.

Foeniculum vulgare – Umbelliferae

Fennel

Like the other members of the *Umbelliferae* family, fennel originates near the Mediterranean, particularly southern Europe. It has since spread around the world.

Benefits

* Good for digestion, flatulence
* Eases general fatigue
* Relieves fluid retention; useful in slimming
* Helps with bladder infections
* Breath freshener; promotes healthy gums
* Treats eye infections

Fennel has been used since ancient times as both a condiment and medicine. In his book of remedies, Hippocrates noted that if fennel was eaten for a few weeks prior to giving birth, it would promote the flow of breast milk. For the Ancient Greeks, fennel was thought of as a diuretic and classified as a slimming herb. In India, the seeds are given at the end of a meal to aid digestion and sweeten breath (especially good after a hot curry).

Top French phytotherapist Dr Belaiche recommended it for anaemia and as a heart tonic, in case of bad circulation. He mentioned its use in convalescence and when one is feeling low or depressed. More recently, Doctors Maury and Leclerc classified fennel as a tonic, stomachic, carminative and emmenagogic (inducing menstruation). It can be used to reduce puffiness in the eyes and can be helpful in the treatment of eye infections.

To obtain the essential oil the seeds are crushed for distillation. The resulting oil is pale yellow in colour. It has an aniseed aroma with camphory, herby notes.

Dangers

The essential oil can cause allergies and irritations in people with sensitive skin. It can also cause headaches. Be cautious and never leave the oil where children might find it. Essential oil of anise is often used to adulterate fennel essential oil.

Gaultheria procumbens – Ericaceae
Wintergreen

Wintergreen originates in the northern USA and Canada. It can grow in mountainous regions as well as on sandy desert plains.

Benefits

* Diuretic: good for cellulite
* Anti-rheumatic
* Stimulant
* Antiseptic
* Emmenagogic (induces menstruation)

There are approximately 200 species of this small evergreen shrub. The shrub has oval, toothed leaves that are crimson above and a very pale green underneath. It produces white drooping flowers and vibrant red berries.

The essential oil is distilled from the leaves and is colourless. With age the oil turns to a reddish-yellow brown and should not be used in this state. The fresh oil has an agreeable aroma – a little vanilla with a peppery note. The main constituent is methyl salicylate (90–95%), an ester responsible for the aroma. To obtain the essential oil, the leaves are macerated in hot water for approximately twenty-four hours.

Wintergreen is well known to the American Indians who embrace its remarkable therapeutic properties. In times of pain and fever the leaves are chewed or made into teas. In the early twentieth century, French doctors prescribed wintergreen for joint and muscle pain. Swain Panacea was an early nineteenth-century remedy containing wintergreen. Used in conjunction with other essential oils, wintergreen can be successful in treating cellulite. It is also a useful diuretic and slimming aid.

Hypericum perforatum – Hypericaceae
Millepertuis

Millepertuis is found near riverbanks, along woody paths and meadows throughout Europe.

Benefits

* Rejuvenating properties
* Helps heal burns and scar tissue
* Good for greasy hair: rebalances sebum secretions
* Helps with age spots on hands
* Treats couperose (prominent veins)
* Helps with insomnia, depressive states
* Good anti-inflammatory agent

Millepertuis is a very common herbaceous perennial with bright yellow flowers that bloom in early June. The name 'millepertuis' means 'thousand holes' because the leaves appear to have been pierced with tiny little holes, more visible when you hold the leaf to the light. These 'holes' are really just the essential oil glands and when you rub the leaf between your fingers they release a slightly bitter incense smell.

In the Middle Ages people thought that the plant would help banish evil spirits if they kept it at home or put a wreath of the flowers outside their door. In the sixteenth century it was believed that the devil hated the smell and would run away from it. Recently millepertuis has made a comeback. In Germany around 60 tonnes of the plant is processed per year for use in the treatment of nervous conditions and insomnia.

The principal constituent of the essential oil is a tannin called hyperine glucoside. It is sometimes referred to as 'nerves arnica' as it is a sedative and is wonderful in treating all nervous disorders. Phytotherapist Dr Leclerc used it successfully in the treatment of burns and scar tissue as it accelerates healing. I have also found it extremely useful for these purposes.

Jasminum officinale – Oleaceae

Jasmine

Jasmine originated in India, China and Persia and its name comes from the Persian *Yasmin*. It appeared in Europe in the mid-1500s where it quickly acclimatized. It also grows well in Israel, Egypt and Lebanon.

Benefits

* Soothes infected eyes
* Helps with the menopause
* Facilitates labour
* Treats insomnia
* Helps depression
* Used in perfume

There are more than 300 species of this hardy, evergreen shrub. It can reach up to 6m (20ft) without support. The leaves are pinnate and of a dark green although there are varieties that have silver-edged leaves. Its flowers have the most exquisite aroma that is so appreciated in the best perfumes as it forms the middle notes (see page 161). The species *J. grandiflorum* is the most common and is almost exclusively cultivated for the perfumery trade. It is also called Spanish jasmine because Spanish sailors brought it back to the Mediterranean from the Far East after being intoxicated by its scent. The ketone jasmone, with its echoes of orange blossom, is responsible for the subtle and delicate aroma of jasmine – no synthetic version can ever match it.

Jasmine flowers are best harvested very early in the morning as they only retain their aroma until the first light of the sun. After picking they need to be quickly distilled otherwise the aroma will be lost. The world's annual production is only about 6 tonnes and it is thus considered one of the most precious oils. Indeed, it is often described as the pearl of essential oils.

In aromatherapy it is difficult to find true essential oil of jasmine. It is replaced by an absolute (an oil that uses solvents in the process, which are often found in the final oil) that is more suitable for use in the perfume industry.

Another variety called Zambak or Arabian jasmine was introduced to Britain in 1690. This is made into garlands and used by Hindus to honour guests. When I visited Bangalore in India I was presented with a jasmine garland and it left such an impression of pure joy and delight and I felt so peaceful that I even slept in it! I learnt later that the flowers are presented to the god Vishnu in Hindu religious ceremonies. According to Ancient Indian texts, jasmine was considered an aphrodisiac because of its spellbinding sweet note. In China jasmine is used to perfume tea.

When sprayed in a room it gives such an uplifting feeling and instantly makes one feel better. It helps to relax the senses and instils confidence, and I love using it for those reasons.

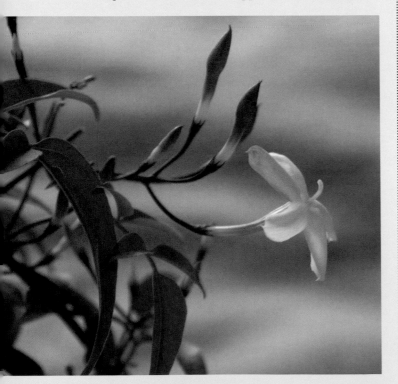

Juniperus communis – Cupressaceae

Juniper

Juniper originated around the Mediterranean regions and in the Middle East, but is now also grown in North America, the Canadian forests, northern Asia and Africa.

Benefits
* Helps with acne and skin problems
* Used as a slimming aid
* Diuretic
* Treats urinary infections
* Eases coughs
* Helps rheumatism
* Treats liver problems
* Antiseptic

There are approximately sixty different species of juniper. Some think the name juniper comes from the Latin *juniores* or 'youth', referring to the new berries that appear constantly on the tree. Others claim that it gets its name from the Celtic word *gen*, meaning small bush. The French call it *genièvre*, the basis of the word gin and the drink made from the berries.

In ancient times, juniper was burnt during religious ceremonies, and in the smallpox epidemic of 1870 it was used in French hospitals as an antiseptic and bactericide. The British kept demons away by burning juniper wood in their homes, while bunches hung above the front door on May eve (the coming of summer) were said to ward off witches. Decoctions of the rejuvenating berries were drunk as an elixir of youth.

The essential oil is obtained by distillation of the black berries; this produces a complex oil that has many antiseptic properties. It is quite safe to apply neat to the skin.

Dangers
Be careful when buying juniper essential oil as sometimes turpentine is used to adulterate it.

Juniperus oxycedrus – Cupressaceae

Cade

This is a small evergreen cedar that grows in the south of France and around the Mediterranean. It is a hardy spreading plant, which can vary in size from a low shrub to a tree of roughly 6m (20ft).

Benefits
* Treats eczema, psoriasis
* Helps hair and scalp problems, alopecia
* Treats herpes

The essential oil of cade is distilled from the dry wood of a mature tree. It is resinous and dark brown in colour with a strong tarry smell that is acrid and bitter. It is very often falsified with different chemicals so in order to identify a true cade oil, you must make sure it is a transparent, reddish colour. If it is adulterated, it will be blackish-brown.

It was first introduced to medicine in the mid-nineteenth century for the treatment of skin diseases and has shown great results, mainly because of its antiseptic properties. It is excellent in the treatment of skin eruptions such as psoriasis, scalp problems (the neat essential oil is one of the best treatments for hair loss and dandruff) and those caused by parasites. It has also been successfully used by vets to treat skin problems in animals.

Dangers
Cade essential oil is very often adulterated so make sure your supply comes from a good source.

Lavandula angustifolia/officinalis – Labiatae

Lavender

Lavender originates from Persia and around the Mediterranean. Most is cultivated in Provence in France, where many thousands of acres are given over to its cultivation. The high altitude combined with the hard and rocky ground is what the plant needs to flourish.

Some small crops are grown in England and even as far away as Tasmania and New Zealand. Lavender used to grow in abundance around the suburbs of London, as evidenced in the name Lavender Hill in Clapham, for example.

Benefits

* Helps heal burns
* Heals wounds
* Antiseptic
* Bactericide, treats acne
* Calms allergies
* Anti-inflammatory
* Fungicide
* Aids bruising
* Soothing, sedative
* Heart tonic
* Helps with irregular periods
* Soothes nervousness and aids anxiety
* Blood cleanser
* Helps with urinary problems
* Brings shine to hair

Lavender has been used in both medicine and perfume since the earliest times. The Romans had baths infused with it (its name comes from the Latin *lavare* meaning 'to wash'). St Hildegarde (1098–1179) mentioned it in her treatise and it was grown in many a monastery garden for its medicinal properties. Charles VI of France reportedly sat on pillows filled with lavender and ladies of the court would sew lavender bags into their skirts.

The oil is pale yellow or yellowy green but falsified oils (cheap versions which are not 100% pure) can turn dark.

The quality of the oil very much depends on the type of soil and the climate in which the lavender is grown. Provençal lavender yields a better-quality essential oil because it has a higher concentration of esters. For this reason it also has a sweeter and fruitier fragrance. Lavender that is grown in the UK has a higher proportion of lineol and therefore smells more of camphor.

There are several different varieties of lavender but the main ones are *L. angustifolia*, *L. vera* (when you see the term '*vera*' attached to lavender this means it's a wild variety) and *L. spica*. The latter, also known as spike or Old English lavender, produces aspic essential oil (see opposite). When aspic and lavender are crossed they produce lavandin essential oil – obtained by steam distillation of this hybrid lavender (see opposite).

Lavender is well known for its ability to heal burns, perhaps due to the famous story involving one of the fathers of aromatherapy, Dr Gattefossé. After badly burning his hand in his lab he mistakenly plunged it into a vat of lavender essential oil. As a result, the wound healed rapidly and the pain stopped. Dr Gattefossé thus classified lavender as a good treatment for burns.

Lavender is wonderful in relaxation and beauty treatments – a few drops added to a bath can restore the spirit when stressed. It can be used with fennel in an oil to help combat cellulite. It brings shine to hair and is wonderful in preparations for acne as it helps normalize gland secretions.

Lavender has so many multiple uses that everyone would benefit from carrying a small bottle around.

Lavender is wonderful in relaxation and beauty treatments — a few drops added to a bath can restore the spirit when stressed.

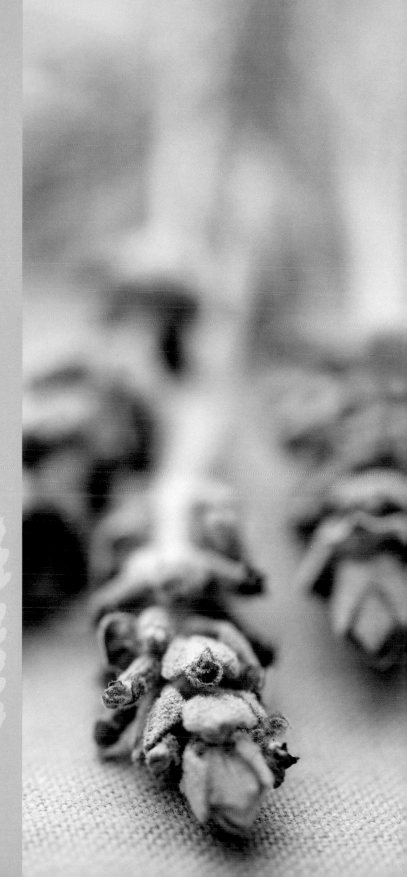

Lavandula fragrans/delphinensis – Labiatae

Lavandin

Lavandin is the most cultivated lavender – mainly in Europe but also Japan and the USA. It first appeared in Provence in 1920 and now makes up over 80% of the lavender grown there. The flowers are a very dark blue (whereas true lavender is a mauvey-grey).

The essential oil of lavandin is much cheaper than lavender and not as therapeutic. It has a large proportion of borneol (40–50%) and camphor, and therefore smells quite acrid. It is normally only used in cosmetics, soap and toiletries.

Lavandula spica – Labiatae

Aspic

Aspic grows at a much lower altitude than true lavender. It smells slightly like rosemary and although not as appreciated as lavender, it is rich in essential oils. Aspic gets its name from spica or spike lavender. Also known as Old English lavender, this variety has been around for centuries and the essential oil was being distilled as early as the seventeenth century. Dr Nicolas Lemery noted that it was good for pain, migraines and as a relaxant. It also has great anti-inflammatory properties and phytotherapist Dr Leclerc found it useful in treating acne as it helps remove infection and heals scar tissue.

In France vets rub aspic on the paws of cats and dogs with rheumatic conditions. It is also rubbed on the backs and legs of horses after long races.

Dangers

The properties of aspic are similar to those of true lavender but, unlike the latter, it can be toxic – its constituents can cause vomiting so it should never be used in large quantities (for example, in the bath).

Melaleuca alternifolia – Myrtaceae

Tea tree

The tea tree originates in Australia and is the only one of the thirty-four species of *Melaleuca* unique to this country. Its main habitat is around New South Wales.

Benefits

* Natural antibiotic
* Disinfectant
* Antiseptic
* Heals scar tissue
* Helps with acne, abscesses and boils
* Treats athlete's foot
* Soothes bites and stings
* Helps impetigo
* Treats ulcers

Tea tree is a small, paperbark tree, only growing to 7m (23ft) in height and is related to cajuput and niaouli (see opposite). It needs humid, swampy soil in order to grow. In the past, this made it difficult to cultivate as deadly snakes and spiders also frequented the areas in which it thrived.

Aborigines have used tea tree as an antiseptic and bactericide for centuries. More recently, many studies have taken place in Australia to prove its antibiotic properties. The results have been amazing and the oil was given to both the Australian Army and Navy in 1939.

Tea tree is such a well-known essential oil that it has appeared in many preparations during the last couple of decades. It is very useful in aromatherapy and it is easy to find everywhere. Tea tree has been used in the treatment of burns, for gynaecological conditions and for ear, nose and throat infections. It is the perfect essential oil to keep in your handbag as you can use it for everything – cuts, burns, spots and as an antiseptic.

The essential oil is distilled from its leaves. It has a camphory, spicy scent and is colourless or pale yellow. Terpenes are the main constituents and it is these that give tea tree its strong anti-bacterial properties.

Melaleuca leucadendron – Myrtaceae

Cajuput

Cajuput originated in the Moluccas, now the East Indies, and can also be found in Vietnam, Malaysia, Indonesia and the north of Australia.

Benefits

* Helps cystitis
* Treats skin problems: acne; dermatitis; eczema
* Helps rheumatic conditions
* Eases respiratory problems, bronchitis
* Helps cases of flu
* Calms headaches

Cajuput is a beautiful tree of approximately 15m (50ft) in height. It has a whitish bark with leaves that are similar to eucalyptus, and small round fruits.

The name cajuput comes from the Malay *caju-puti* meaning 'white tree'. When I was living in Malaysia I found that, mixed with other essential oils, it was good in the treatment of cold and flu symptoms, viral infections and coughs. For this I would suggest diffusing the oil in a room to rid it of infection.

The essential oil is a very pale greenish colour with principal constituents of cineol, eucalyptol, pinene and terpinol – all good for the respiratory system. It is distilled from the young twigs, leaves and buds, and has a camphory, spicy smell with a hint of pine.

Dr G. Guibourt mentioned it in his 1876 book *The Natural History of Simple Drugs*, prescribing it for use in the treatment of infections of the urinary system, intestinal problems and cystitis. Cajuput's antiseptic properties help soothe acne and it also calms headaches.

Dangers

Cajuput should only be used externally. Be warned that it is often adulterated with turpentine.

Melaleuca viridiflora – Myrtaceae

Niaouli

Melaleuca viridiflora is closely related to cajuput and grows principally in New Caledonia and Australia.

Benefits

* Antiseptic
* Bactericide
* Helps dermatitis
* Treats stings and bites
* Anti-inflammatory
* Calms headaches, fevers
* Helps cystitis and urinary problems
* Treats rheumatic conditions
* Aids cicatrization (healing)

Niaouli is an evergreen tree with extremely aromatic leaves. The essential oil is obtained from the distillation of the leaves and twigs. Another name for the oil is 'gomen' as many years ago the distillation took place near the port of Gomen in New Caledonia. It was highly valued by the locals who used it to treat fevers, rheumatic conditions and as a way of healing scars and wounds.

The principal constituent of the oil is eucalyptol (50–60%) and its aroma is very similar to that of eucalyptus – very fresh and balsamic. It is pale yellow in colour but can also be a dark yellow, depending on its provenance.

Niaouli is an evergreen tree with extremely aromatic leaves ... used to treat fevers, rheumatic conditions and as a way of healing scars and wounds.

Melissa officinalis – Labiatae

Melissa

Melissa originated in Asia and the Middle East but it is now also cultivated in France, Spain, Germany and North America.

Benefits

* Helps acne, reduces chicken pox marks
* Aids cicatrization (healing)
* Calming
* Good for depression and stress
* Helps with PMS and menopausal problems

Melissa grows like a little bush and can reach a height of 30–70cm (1–2ft). Its leaves have a lacy edge and the plant's whitish flowers bloom in Europe from early June to early September.

Melissa was the name of a Greek nymph who was turned into a bee by Zeus. In fact, the name Melissa comes from the Greek word for honeybee. In the European *Pharmaocopea* it is prescribed for stress, anxiety, insomnia and nervous disorders. Nowadays it is used to treat symptoms of stress, depression, heart problems, respiratory problems and digestive disorders. I have prescribed it many times, especially for stressed-out city workers.

Melissa is also known as 'bee's pimento' in France and some think that it even has a cheering effect on the bees after they take its nectar! Interestingly, it is also useful if you happen to get stung by a bee – just crush some of the leaves and rub them onto the sting. Melissa is one of the most expensive essential oils to produce. Be aware of this when you want to buy it, as cheaper versions will not provide the same curative properties.

Dangers

Be sure to buy pure oil – it can often be falsified with lemongrass, which will make it quite yellow in colour. Never take it internally.

Mentha piperita – Labiatae

Peppermint/Mint

Mint is cultivated in Europe, the USA, Japan and Chile.

Benefits

* Anti-ageing
* Detoxifier
* Helps congested skin, spots, acne
* Antiseptic and bactericide
* Tonic for the circulation, heart, blood
* Good for muscular cramps
* Aids digestion
* Analgesic
* Promotes mouth and teeth health
* Helps hot flushes, headaches, migraines

Peppermint is most commonly used in tisanes and cooking but it has an important place in aromatherapy too. Because of its phenol content, the oil is a wonderful bactericide and is great in the treatment of spots and acne, bruising and swellings. Its analgesic properties help to mask pain and it has a cooling effect on the symptoms of headaches, migraines and hot flushes.

There are over twenty species of mint and, as a result, many hybrids are found around the world. *M. piperita* is the variety used in therapy. The plant is shiny and dark green with reddish flowers that appear at the end of the twiggy stems. The oil itself has a hot, peppery, camphory smell. It is strong and refreshing, and highly balsamic.

'Mitcham mint' is cultivated around Europe and its oil is highly appreciated. Peppermint from Japan contains more camphrene; it is heavier and not always agreeable to the nose. This variety is used mostly for the extraction of menthol.

Dangers

Never use the essential oil in the bath; the cooling action of the menthol could cause problems with blood pressure.

Myristica fragrans – Myristicaceae

Nutmeg

Nutmeg is cultivated in the East Indies, Malaysia, Sumatra and French Guinea. It was first introduced to Asia by the Arabs.

Benefits

* Helps with pre-menstrual pain
* Intestinal antiseptic
* Good for symptoms of flu and bronchitis
* Aids digestion and eases flatulence
* Helps rheumatic conditions, cricked neck, general aches and pains
* Tonic for stress and fatigue
* Slightly analgesic
* Helps blood circulation
* Helps sexual fatigue, lack of interest

Nutmeg trees are known as 'harem trees' because in order to produce fruit, only one male tree is needed per twenty females.

When I lived in Malaysia in the 1970s, I was fortunate enough to have a sweet-smelling nutmeg tree growing in my garden. The bark was very smooth and greenish-brown in colour, and the tree itself was over 12m (40ft) in height.

The fresh fruit is a brilliant red but soon wrinkles with age – the fruit itself is known as mace, while the seed inside is the actual nutmeg. The fruits are gathered two or three times a year and are dried in the sun. They are then split open and the nutmeg is removed, crushed and steam-distilled to produce the essential oil. This smells superb – warm and aromatic, with bitter, peppery notes. It is colourless and fluid but will thicken with age.

In 1569, Dr Fernal described nutmeg as the greatest stimulant to the nervous system – grated in food and used internally, and the oil applied externally. The eighteenth-century French *Treatise of Medicine* devoted a large entry to nutmeg and included twenty-eight recipes containing it! French researcher Pulligny famously wrote a book with over 800 pages dedicated to the nutmeg tree and the spice. It has even been found effective for foot massage during labour (it can hasten contractions). It is used in many tonics and to flavour liqueurs, and can conceal the bad taste of many other medicines.

Essential oil of nutmeg is a wonderful tonic and I have given it to many of my patients for the treatment of stress and general fatigue. Rubbing the torso with oil made from nutmeg and a carrier oil can ease the symptoms of flu and bronchitis. This also works as a remedy for sporting injuries and cricked necks. Follow with a hot compress. A French medicinal book by Dr Valnet in the 1960s prescribed nutmeg as a perfect remedy for male sexual problems as it reportedly arouses desire.

Dangers

The principal constituent is myristicine, which is a strong tonic and stimulant – use it carefully. However, it is also toxic in large doses and can cause nausea and quicken the heartbeat. For this reason, the oil should only be used in small doses and never in pregnancy. The School of Salerno (the fifteenth-century 'Regiment of Health') noted that 'one nut is good, another is less good, the third kills'.

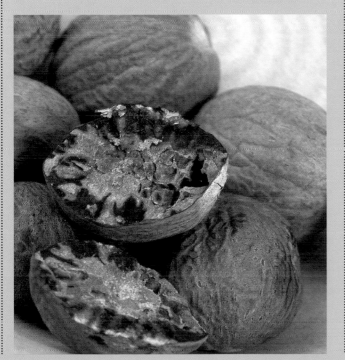

Nardostachys jatamansi – Valerianaceae

Spikenard

Spikenard is native to India and grows near rivers and mountains, sometimes reaching quite an altitude with its scent changing accordingly.

Benefits
* Helps eczema
* Treats skin eruptions
* Anti-bacterial properties
* Soothing, especially in pregnancy

Related to valerian, spikenard is one of the oldest oils. It is well known in India but not so well known in Europe, but if you have the opportunity to smell it – do, it is an experience! In his treatise, the Greek physician Discorides said that it smelt of goat, but I prefer to relate it to moss and fallen autumn leaves. It's a unique plant, partly due to its blooming rhizomes (the underground stems that are crushed to produce the amber-coloured essential oil).

Spikenard has been mentioned in ancient scripts and was part of the ointment of sweet spices with which Mary Magdalen anointed Christ's feet.

When I was in India I was told that spikenard is used to treat old injuries and pains, and to correct the flow of energy and relieve tension – perfect for the stresses of the twenty-first century. A yogi told me that spikenard is used a lot in combination with yoga as it activates energy and is good when rubbed on the lower part of the back. It also has cooling anti-bacterial and anti-fungal properties and can help in the treatment of eczema and skin eruptions. It is now used in decoctions and tisanes – as a root tea, it can help a woman have a happy pregnancy.

Ocimum spp. – Labiatae

Basil

There are around 150 varieties of basil, of different colours with different leaves and flowers; some even have different constituents. The common variety, however, originates in India but is now cultivated throughout the Mediterranean, Java, the Seychelles, Florida and Réunion. The common plant grows up to 50cm (20 inches) and has white flowers with dark green leaves that smell wonderful if bruised.

Benefits

* Helps headaches, migraines
* Aids colds, flu
* Helps with digestive troubles
* Good for insomnia
* Aids anxiety, nervous tension
* Antiseptic
* Anti-spasmodic and relaxant
* Pick-me-up
* Aids PMS and irregular periods
* Rejuvenating

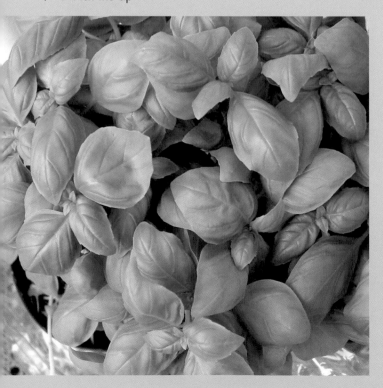

The Romans mentioned basil as both a medicinal and a culinary herb. Pliny recommended it against jaundice, as a diuretic and as an aphrodisiac. In AD 10 Arab doctors claimed that the lemony aroma of basil could help migraines, problems of the nervous system and could improve breathing by cleansing the respiratory system. They smoked the dried herb with tobacco to give them a mental kick and also powdered it to make snuff to cure headaches and colds.

Phytotherapist Dr Leclerc prescribed basil as a general tonic for the nervous system, for nervous dyspepsia, to calm gastric spasms, for general fatigue after illness and anxiety.

Basil has been nicknamed 'the magic herb' as it has so many different uses, and even today it is used in everything from pasta sauce to perfume. It has found its place as a super remedy in the twenty-first century. It is an effective intestinal antiseptic and helps to rejuvenate the whole body. It is wonderful for all stress-related problems and I have found it so useful in many face and body skin-care treatments. If you can't get hold of the essential oil, use the fresh leaves regularly in your cooking.

In preparations, the essential oil mixes well with lavender, clary sage, lemon, patchouli and marjoram.

Dangers

One of the constituents of basil, estragol (or methyl chavicol) can be quite toxic for people with sensitive skin so it's always advisable to mix it with other essential oils. Do not apply neat to the skin.

Basil has been nicknamed 'the magic herb' as it has so many different uses, and even today it is used in everything from pasta sauce to perfume.

Origanum majorana – Labiatae

Marjoram

Marjoram originates in Asia but is also cultivated in Spain, North Africa and Hungary.

Benefits

* Helps stress and eases nervous tension
* Anti-ageing effect on wrinkles; facial muscles relax as a result of using the oil
* Calms headaches, migraine
* Sedative action for insomnia

Marjoram is a small, vivacious plant growing from 30–60cm (1–2ft). It has white and purple flowers and a strong aromatic smell. Common in France, marjoram is well known and appreciated there. It has lots of culinary uses and is a mainstay of many dishes.

Marjoram was known to the Ancient Egyptians who used it in prayers to the god of the dead, Osiris. The Ancient Greeks saw it as a symbol of love and fidelity and wove it into crowns to give to newly-married couples. Dioscorides prescribed a marjoram balm for nervous tension and advised his patients to apply it to their temples and solar plexus. Lotions were made for hair to help it retain its lustre and shine. It was described as an antispasmodic and expectorant by the School of Salerno who gave it to pregnant women in order to facilitate labour. It would ease contractions and calm the pain. In the Renaissance, marjoram was said to combat infection.

The essential oil is high in phenols (80% is comprised of carvocrol and thymol), which have antiseptic properties and are strong stimulants for the immune system. The essential oil has a peppery, herby scent with a hint of pine.

Dangers

Avoid using marjoram on young children as it is too strong a stimulant.

Origanum vulgare – Labiatae

Oregano

Oregano grows wild throughout Europe and Asia.

Benefits

* Anti-ageing
* Anti-fatigue
* Antiseptic and anti-viral
* Helps eczema, psoriasis, burns
* Tonic for the nervous system
* Helps respiratory system
* Aids general fatigue and convalescence

Oregano is often called wild marjoram and like all the members of the *Labiatae* family, it has multiple uses and properties. The plant has pinkish/purple flowers and when you rub the leaves in your hand it exudes a strong aroma.

Ancient writers Hippocrates, Dioscorides and Pliny mentioned oregano in their work. It was indispensable in the treatment of respiratory and digestive problems, and was reputed to have carminative and warming properties. In an 1837 treatise, *Traité des Plantes Usuelles*, Dr Roques recorded its power in treating viruses and prescribed aromatic oregano baths and lotions to his patients. Essential oil of oregano is renowned for its antiseptic and bactericide properties. Research and aromatograms (ways of discovering constituents within an essential oil) have shown oregano to be extremely effective in fighting many viruses such as *streptococcus* and *candida albicans*.

Oregano is wonderful in the treatment of skin problems such as eczema, psoriasis and general scar tissue. It can also be used to stimulate the healing of burns and other wounds.

The oil itself is dark to light brown in colour with a strong pine-like smell, spicy, bitter and warm.

Dangers

Never use essential oil of oregano neat – it must always be diluted with wheatgerm or other emollient oils.

Pelargonium spp. – Geraniaceae

Geranium

The geranium plant is cultivated in Réunion, South Africa, Madagascar, Egypt and Congo. Species are also found in China, India and Russia. The climate and quality of the soil are vital factors in the production of the essential oil, but I believe that Réunion's geranium Bourbon is by far the best.

Benefits

❋ Helps with dermatitis, skin rashes

❋ Good for burns, cuts, insect bites

❋ Aids throat infections, colds and flu

❋ Treats athlete's foot, chilblains

❋ Helps eye infections

❋ Soothes itchy scalp

❋ Helps with anxiety/stress

❋ Room disinfectant

❋ Helps with PMS and menopausal problems

❋ Sedative

❋ Nerve tonic

❋ Antiseptic

❋ Bactericide

The word *pelargonium* comes from the Greek *pelargos* or stork because the fruit has a resemblance to the neck of the bird. *Graveolens* (the rose-scented geranium) means strong, persistent aroma. In ancient times the geranium represented sexual maturity and the flowers were worn as a way of indicating this fact to a partner.

There are over 200 species recognized, but only *P. graveolens*, *P. roseum*, *P. odoratissimum*, *P. capitatum* and *P. radula* are used in therapy. (It's important to remember that these are completely different to the species on our windowsills!) Flowers and leaves are picked before they come into bloom. It takes over 300kg (660lb) to make just 1kg (2¼lb) of essential oil. Distillation of the essential oil in the perfume industry began in the seventeenth century.

In 1847, the French physician Dermason led research into the best varieties of geranium with which to produce a top-quality essential oil. It was during this research that the therapeutic properties of geranium came to light.

According to Dr Sarbach, who conducted research into the antiseptic properties of essential oils in the 1960s, essential oil of geranium takes approximately sixty to eighty minutes (depending on the weight of a person) to absorb into the skin.

Geranium is one of my absolute favourite essential oils. It was introduced to me by Marguerite Maury, who used it for treating many skin conditions – its healing power results in a radiant glow. She also loved it for its wonderful aroma, fresh and floral at the same time, with notes of mint and rose, and praised its power in treating a wide range of different medical problems.

For a simple pick-me-up, put two drops of geranium oil onto the palm of your hand and rub in vigorously for a few moments. Cup your nose with your palms and breathe in the soothing vapours. It has such a good effect in rebalancing the emotions in times of stress and anxiety, helping you to relax – try applying it neat on your solar plexus before yoga or other exercise. It is great for circulation and you will find that chilblains get better overnight after rubbing with it. It brings a radiant glow to the face and it can be very effective for women going through the menopause. Geranium is also great in the winter months – its antiseptic properties can help banish colds and flu. It is good inhaled with other essential oils as it can reinforce their action. Geranium mixes well with rosemary, lavender, lemon and chamomile.

Dangers

Geranium is sometimes falsified with cedarwood, lemongrass or turpentine and sometimes even artificial esters – these can be easily detected, as they don't dissolve in alcohol. The essential oil is quite expensive so check out the quality before you buy to make sure it is genuine.

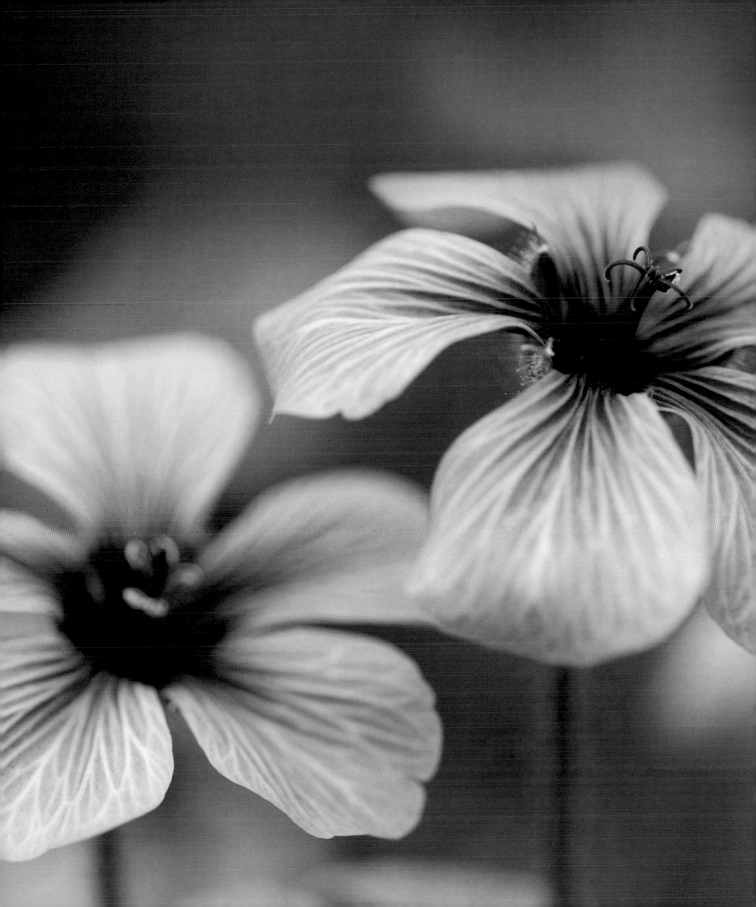

Petroselinum sativum/crispum – Umbelliferae

Parsley

Parsley is native to the eastern Mediterranean but is thought to have originated in Sardinia. It was introduced to northern Europe by the Romans.

Benefits

* Reduces couperose, thread veins, skin irritations
* Helps with PMS and menopausal problems
* Eases cystitis
* Soothes sore eyes
* Diuretic
* Treats circulation problems

There are many different varieties of parsley but all have the same edible carrot-shaped roots. The common types have dark green leaves with pale yellow-green flowers that grow in umbels.

Both the Ancient Greeks and Romans used parsley. Victorious Greek soldiers were crowned with parsley as a symbol of vigour and strength. Pliny and Greek physician Galen said that no sauce or salad should be without it. They considered it to be a diuretic, emmenagogic (inducing menstruation) and as a treatment for kidney stones. King Charlemagne ordered parsley to be grown in the royal vegetable gardens.

Research carried out on the diuretic and emmenagogic properties of its constituent apiol by two scientists, Jovet and Homelle in 1850, found that apiol acts on both the nervous and circulatory systems. Apiol also helps to regulate the menstrual cycle and calm pain.

As a beauty treatment, essential oil of parsley has a calming action on blotchy and irritated skin. It also helps in the treatment of thread veins and skin irritations.

Dangers

Parsley must be carefully dosed as in large quantities the essential oil can have the opposite effect to that desired. Symptoms sometimes felt are dizziness, low blood pressure and it has even been implicated in miscarriage.

Pimpinella anisum – Umbelliferae

Anise

Anise originally comes from the Orient but is also grown around the Mediterranean – especially Egypt and the Middle East.

Benefits

* Digestive aid
* Helps with anxiety and nervousness, nervous palpitations
* Aids relaxation
* Eases asthmatic conditions
* Helps with PMS and menopausal problems
* Sedative

Also known as aniseed or sweet cumin, anise is related to dill, caraway and fennel. The essential oil can often be falsified with fennel and caraway. The hot, dry climate in which it grows gives it a stronger perfume and taste. It has feathery leaves and yellowish-white flowers and grows up to about 60cm (2ft) high.

The Romans introduced anise to Europe, adding the seeds to bread as an aid to digestion. Pliny wrote much about the benefits of using aniseeds and advised on drinking aniseed tea before bed, as it is a good sedative. He also mentioned its uses in skin-care and recommended that women add it to skin lotions in order to retain their youthful looks!

In medieval France anise was recommended as an aid to meditation and as a calming medicine for the nervous system. In India, aniseeds are used instinctively after a meal to prevent indigestion and chewing the seeds slowly helps prevent flatulence and hiccups.

In France, anise is used (under strict controls) to

In India, aniseeds are used instinctively after a meal to prevent indigestion and chewing the seeds slowly helps prevent flatulence and hiccups.

flavour toothpastes and mouthwashes, and seeds are sometimes fed to cows to stimulate milk production. It is also a favourite in the drinks Pastis and Ricard.

Dangers

Essential oil of anise is very poisonous and can cause numbness of the muscles followed by paralysis. The high percentage of anethol combined with methyl chavicol in the oil can be tremendously toxic, so it should not be used in therapy or sold to the public. The oil should only be used by an experienced practitioner and, because of this, it is strictly controlled. It is still an important plant, however, for the reasons stated above.

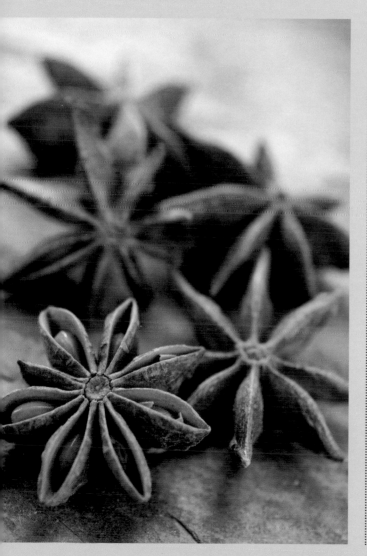

Pinus sylvestris – Coniferae

Pine

The pine tree is native to Europe, Russia and North America.

Benefits

✳ Helps with skin eruptions, acne, spots
✳ Eases respiratory problems
✳ Helps with PMS
✳ Treats urinary infections
✳ Treats itchy scalp
✳ Reduces inflammation

The most widespread species of pine is the Scots pine, which can grow happily in temperatures as low as -40ºC – it even survived the Ice Age! Pine trees can grow as high as 36m (120ft); they have short, spiky needles and the cones are fully matured after approximately two years.

In the UK, pine kernels have been found in excavations near Roman buildings. 'Father of Medicine' Hippocrates prescribed pine for throat and pulmonary infections and Roman writer Pliny the Elder echoed its properties in his *Natural History*. It is used today in many cases of bronchitis, asthma and pneumonia, and is very effective for cystitis and other urinary infections. Pine oil can soothe an itchy scalp and is great for rheumatic problems. Pine kernels are also rich in nutrients and are delicious in pasta dishes and pesto sauces.

Both the resin and the needles of the pine tree are used in the production of the essential oil. There are over 150 varieties but I prefer the oil that comes from the needles of trees found in Scandinavia and Russia. The essence has a lovely balsamic smell with camphory notes.

Dangers

The essential oil can often be adulterated with turpentine so make sure you buy your oil from a good source.

Piper nigrum – Piperaceae

Black pepper

The black pepper is a creeping vine that is found in Java, Sumatra, India, China and Madagascar.

Benefits

* ✳ Rejuvenating
* ✳ Hastens recovery from cosmetic surgery: overcomes numbness and neuralgia; repairs and restores
* ✳ Stimulates circulation
* ✳ Lowers blood pressure
* ✳ Helps with sports injuries
* ✳ Analgesic
* ✳ Aphrodisiac
* ✳ Tonic for the stomach, digestive
* ✳ Used in perfume

There are more than 900 species of *Piperaceae* but only about ten are used as a spice or for medical purposes. It is a creeping vine that can grow up to 6m (20ft) (for cultivation, it is kept to a more modest 3–3.5m/10–12ft). The vine has beautiful green leaves that grow in abundance and each vine can produce up to 2kg (4lb) peppercorns annually. The peppercorns are picked when green and are then left to dry in the sun where they blacken.

Pliny recorded black pepper as being 'more expensive than gold' and it was mentioned in Chinese and Sanskrit texts from the tenth century BC. In Chinese medicine it was considered to be a 'yang' (hot) ingredient. It the Middle Ages it was so precious that members of royalty would receive tributes in peppercorns.

I have combined it with other essential oils to accelerate its warming and dynamizing effects – black pepper intensifies the smell of rose essential oil for example, and if you add it to rosemary, you get an oil that is wonderfully warming. For these reasons it is very useful in the perfume industry as it reinforces the aroma of flowers. Black pepper essential oil contains piperine, which can be copied synthetically and unfortunately it is piperine that is more often used (see 'Dangers', below).

For patients recovering after cosmetic surgery I have prescribed remedies that include black pepper. It is great for warming up the facial muscles and stimulating the circulation, helping to overcome numbness and regain feeling. It is a wonderful essence for repairing and reconstructing.

The first recorded distillation of the essential oil took place in the sixteenth century. It is yellow-green in colour and I love its spicy, hot, piquant aroma. The oil is a key ingredient of many warming rubs sold in chemists. Peppercorns aid digestion and I consider them to be the number one spice. I often grind black pepper over berries or fruit compotes – delicious! On a cold day, black pepper can also be added to hot drinks to help warm you up.

Another variety of pepper, *P. cubeda* comes from Indonesia. This essential oil is yellow in colour but more camphory in smell than *P. nigrum* and is not so useful in therapy.

Dangers

One of the constituents of pepper, piperine, is a stimulant alkaloid so precautions should be taken in using it. Only ever use the oil in small quantities as it can cause burns and dermatitis. (Note, however, that, in small quantities, it has good results in the treatment of dermatitis.) Never use on sensitive or pale skins. Do not use if you are asthmatic.

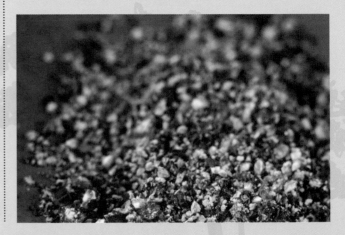

Pogostemon cablin – Umbelliferae

Patchouli

Patchouli essential oil is obtained from a herbaceous shrub called *cablan* that is native to Malaysia. It is now cultivated in many countries including China, Japan and India, where it goes by the name of *patcha* or *patchapat*. Sumatra is the largest producer of the essential oil with China in second place.

Benefits

* Antiseptic
* Prevents ageing spots on hands
* Treats greasy hair
* Helps with all skin problems: acne; dermatitis; psoriasis; burns; heat rash
* Rejuvenates the skin
* Helps with emotional problems
* Used in perfume

When the leaves of the *cablan* plant are rubbed the woody, earthy smell of patchouli is released. The flowers are a whitish-mauve and quite pretty.

Patchouli has always played a great part in traditional Chinese and Japanese medicine. It was used as a stimulant, stomachic and known as a bactericide and antiseptic. In Saudi Arabia it is considered effective in the treatment of fevers, epidemics and many other illnesses – it is wonderful for the immune system.

Its aroma is also highly esteemed and in the 1970s its characteristic scent was used in many perfumes. The 'hippy' culture adopted it and it became a signature scent.

Referred to as 'the friend of the skin', patchouli essential oil helps all manner of skin problems. It refines, tones, strengthens and firms the muscles in the face. It is great for treating acne, dermatitis, psoriasis, burns and heat rash.

I have composed a perfume called '70s' with notes of patchouli to mark this time.

Referred to as 'the friend of the skin', patchouli essential oil helps all manner of skin problems. It refines, tones, strengthens and firms the muscles in the face. It is great for treating acne, dermatitis, psoriasis, burns and heat rash. It has the double action of rehydrating and rebalancing the skin at the same time. Its constituent patchouline makes the oil a good anti-inflammatory and antiseptic.

In 1922, research was carried out by two Italian scientists Gatti and Cayola, on the bactericide and antiseptic properties of patchouli. This was followed in 1962 by more tests by R. Sarbach, which proved the strong antiseptic properties of patchouli.

The principal constituents of the essential oil are patchoulol and sesquiterpenes. There is up to 40% patchouli camphor in the dried leaves, which gives the oil its distinctive aroma.

Dangers

Make sure you buy pure essential oil of patchouli as it can be synthetically produced.

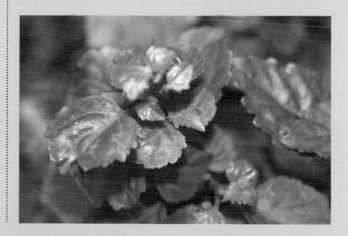

Rosa spp. – Rosaceae

Rose

The rose is cultivated all over the world but originated in the Orient. The most beneficial rose oil comes from either Turkey or Bulgaria. The petals are best picked before a storm and my distillers always know when one is coming because the fragrance from the roses becomes more intense at that time.

Benefits

❋ Helps with PMS and menopausal problems
❋ Helps anorexia and improves appetite
❋ Eases respiratory problems
❋ Soothes sore throats
❋ Helps eye infections
❋ Helps nervous system
❋ Aids insomnia
❋ Helps with depression
❋ Smoothes wrinkles
❋ Anti-ageing
❋ Helps with skin problems
❋ Used in perfume

The history of the rose is almost as old as the world itself. Called the 'queen of flowers', it is a magical plant with an exquisite perfume. There are around 250 species, but thousands more varieties, however only thirty of them come under the 'odorata' (scented) umbrella. From these, only three are cultivated for their perfume.

R. gallica is the first and most abundant. Also called 'French rose' or 'rose of Anatolia', it originated in the Caucasus. The second is *R. centifolia*. Originally Persian, it is also known as the 'rose of Ispahan'. The third is *R. damascena* or the damask rose. Perhaps the most famous, this species originated in Syria and is renowned for its scent (therapeutically it is also the most esteemed).

Another rose also exists; this is rose de mai, a hybrid of *R. gallica* and *R. centifolia*. Only a small quantity is cultivated in Grasse in the south of France to satisfy the tourist industry.

The rose is said to be the emblem of silence – Cupid supposedly gave the god of silence the flower in order to bribe him not to reveal the loves of Venus. This is the reason why many ceilings in dining rooms have 'roses' in their centre. This relates to the old custom of hanging them over the dinner table to ensure that any conversation would be kept in the strictest confidence.

When archaeologist Howard Carter first entered the Egyptian king Tutankhamun's tomb he noticed many bouquets of roses placed next to the mummy. The king's wife, Queen Ankhesenamun, had put them there in order to welcome him into the new world. Even in Ancient Egyptian times, roses were held in high regard.

The Romans thought that wearing roses would protect them from drunkenness and in Ancient Greece Sappho hailed it as the queen of flowers. Also, it was grown for medicinal purposes in the Middle Ages.

The Arab doctor Avicenna gave his patients suffering with blood and respiratory problems a rose jam called zuccar. Rose jam or 'gul' is still used in Turkey today to accompany roast lamb. Some farmers in Turkey also feed their cows rose petals left over from the essential-oil distillation process. As a result the milk tastes of roses!

Essential oil of rose is obtained by the distillation of the petals – you need about 2–3 tonnes of petals to make just 1kg (2¼lb) of essential oil. When I produced moisturizing creams for the High Street, sales consultants couldn't believe that it took at least a thousand rose petals to produce each jar of cream! The essential oil is a pale, yellowy-green in colour and most of the precious oil comes from the petals.

The rose is said to be the emblem of silence — Cupid supposedly gave the god of silence the flower in order to bribe him not to reveal the loves of Venus.

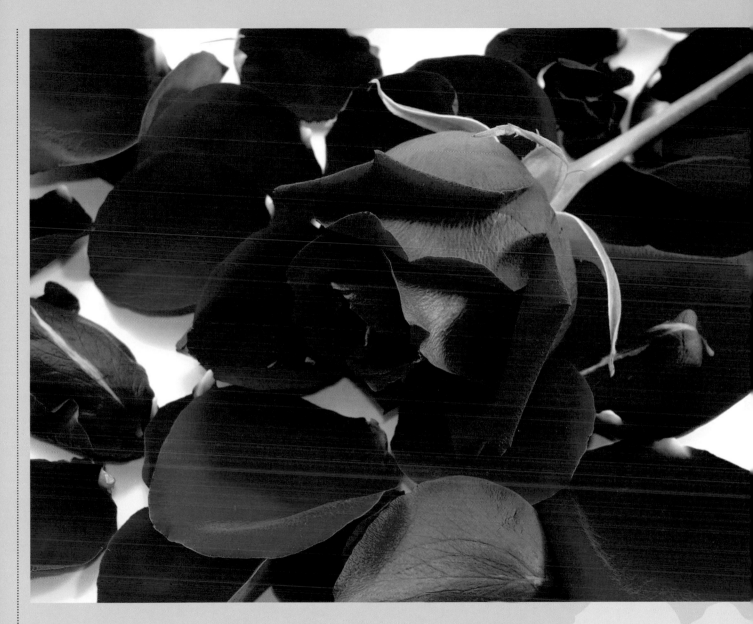

Marguerite Maury advised me to use essential oil of rose on a patient with bad eyesight and a weak heart. She also recommended its use in treating post-natal depression, menstrual problems and calming feelings of anger and fear. It is useful in the treatment of anorexia and helping a person to regain appetite. Some doctors have also talked about its anti-cancer properties and, as a result, have prescribed it for external use. I find that the essential oil has strong rejuvenating skin properties and it is especially useful before and after cosmetic surgery. (It has a high proportion of gammalinolenic acid, which helps the healing of skin tissue.) Wrinkles and broken capillaries also respond well to rose essential oil. It is one of my favourite essential oils to use and will always appear in my preparations, because it is so useful for many ailments.

In beauty, roses were used in the first perfume, 'Hungary water' (named for a fourteenth-century queen of Hungary), and the Ancient Greek physician Galen used essential oil of rose in his recipe for one of the first cold creams.

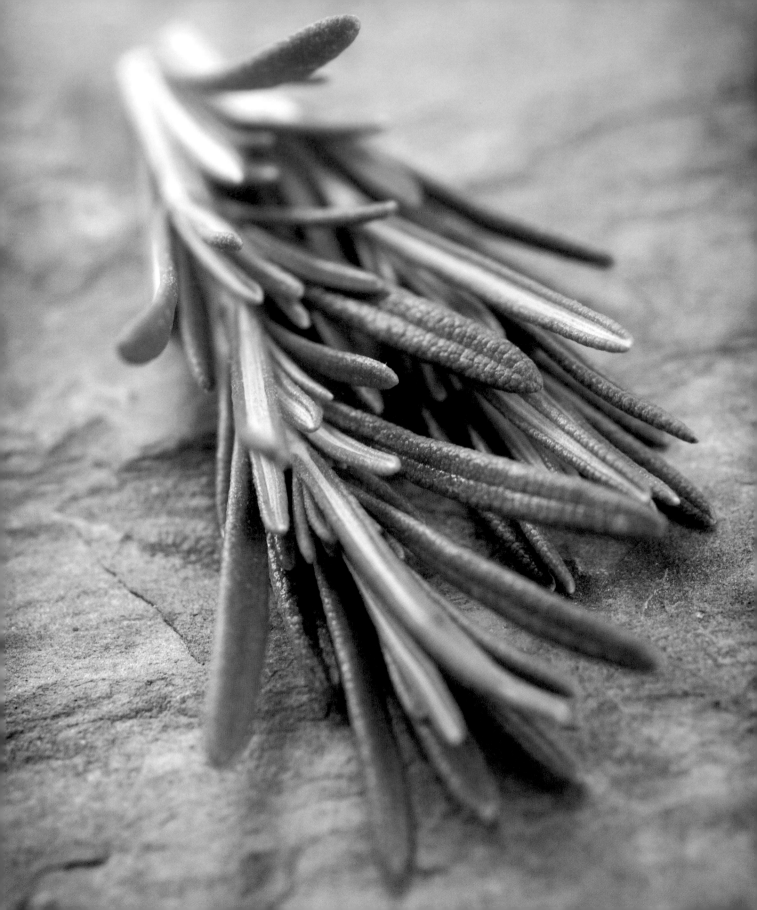

Rosemarinus officinalis – Labiatae

Rosemary

Rosemary is a native of the warm countries of the Mediterranean and North Africa, and has an aversion to the cold.

Benefits

❋ Skin cleanser (good for acne, oily skin, skin infections etc.)
❋ Smoothes wrinkles
❋ Helps with greasy hair, alopecia, as a conditioner for brown hair
❋ Eases depression
❋ Helps with treating rheumatic conditions, gout, aches and pains
❋ Helps with loss of libido
❋ Tonic for the nervous system
❋ Natural antibiotic
❋ Helps with respiratory problems
❋ Blood cleanser
❋ Eases symptoms of food poisoning

The Latin name *rosemarinus* means 'dew of the sea' and it is often found near the coast. Rosemary has small, pale grey–violet flowers with dark centres. Its aroma is very incense-like with a note of camphor and can be released by crushing the leaves in your hand. It is one of the most important essential oils so always keep it to hand.

In ancient times rosemary was used in place of the more expensive frankincense, which had to be imported from Arabia. It was burnt in many religious ceremonies for its incense-like aroma.

It was considered a magic plant by the Greeks and Romans who gave it to their loved ones – my grandmother gave me a bouquet of rosemary and white roses on my wedding day to wish me good luck in my new life. It was also used at funerals as it was said to be a symbol of rebirth. The Roman poet Horace called it a

A key ingredient in the first commercial skin lotion.

magic herb and composed poems in its honour. Before a fight, Roman gladiators rubbed their torsos with rosemary as a way of masking their fear and preparing them for battle. Ancient Greek physician Dioscorides recommended it in treating liver and stomach infections. He even prescribed it as a remedy for weak sight.

The Arabs used rosemary frequently in medicine and were the first to succeed in obtaining its essential oil by distillation.

In Spain it is known as the 'pilgrim's flower' because it was said that during the flight into Egypt, the Virgin Mary sought shelter under a rosemary bush. Since then, rosemary has usually blossomed at Easter. The eighteenth-century French writer Madame de Sevigne said that she couldn't live without a bottle of rosemary in her pocket: just a little sniff for the perfect pick-me-up.

Rosemary, with rose, was one of the main ingredients of the first perfume. 'Hungary water' was so named because it reputedly gave a fourteenth-century queen of Hungary newfound youth at the age of 72. In fact, it worked so well that she ended up marrying the king of Poland.

The best essential oil of rosemary comes from the flowering tops of the bush. The oil is usually colourless but can sometimes be pale yellow to greenish. The percentage of the constituent borneol is high, so rosemary is excellent in treating rheumatic conditions, gout and aches and pains. The constituent phenol also makes it a strong antiseptic. Rosemary tea can help the symptoms of food poisoning, while added to salt it makes a wonderful digestive aid. It is also a great tonic and conditioner for hair, especially brown, and was a key ingredient in the first commercial skin lotion, sold in seventeenth-century Britain.

Dangers

Rosemary can often be adulterated with turpentine, sage and aspic. Always check its provenance. It is not recommended in pregnancy. It can sometimes cause digestive troubles if taken in excess.

Salvia officinalis/Salvia sclarea – Labiatae

Sage/Clary sage

Sage originates in southern Europe. The oil is distilled in France but is also cultivated in Russia.

Benefits

* Regulates sebum secretions
* Helps eczema
* Calms headaches
* Treats excessive sweating
* Anti-rheumatic
* Antiseptic
* Diuretic
* Used in hair treatments
* Helps fatigue and stress
* Astringent
* Helps painful periods

In the Middle Ages the first-ever medical school, the School of Salerno in Naples, recorded an aphorism that sums up the properties of sage – 'How can a man die who has sage growing in his garden?' The name sage comes from the Latin *salvere* meaning 'to save', and folklore mentions 'a plant that heals and saves'.

Sage and clary sage belong to a genus of over 450 species. The plant is hardy and evergreen with pretty little flowers of a light blue, purple for sage, and blue-white for those of clary sage. It can grow to a height of just under 1m (3ft) and grows well next to roses. (It may be because of the essential oils in sage but the plants complement each other.)

Clary sage variety (*S. sclarea*) gets its name from 'clarity' or 'clear' and it is used in many preparations to soothe sore eyes and is highly valued in eye treatments. Clary sage essential oil is a pale yellow colour with an aromatic, camphory fragrance. The main constituents are linalool and linalyl acetate (thujone should not appear).

The seeds were also used for inflammations, swellings of the skin and hay fever. In 1938, Russian biologists recognized the healing properties of the plant and recommended it for women's problems including menopause, menstruation and hot flushes. These properties were echoed by French doctors Valnet, Leclerc and Bélaiche who have written of its sudorific (causing perspiration), blood cleansing, anti-oxidant and antiseptic properties.

Essential oil of sage is pale yellow-green in colour. Its principal constituents are borneol and camphor, but it also has a high thujone content (a constituent not present in clary sage). Thujone can cause skin irritation and allergic reactions so, sage oil must be used with caution and should never be taken internally.

Both sage and clary sage are good fixatives in perfume. Pregnant women may find a sage tea helpful in promoting tranquillity and balancing hormones at the beginning of pregnancy.

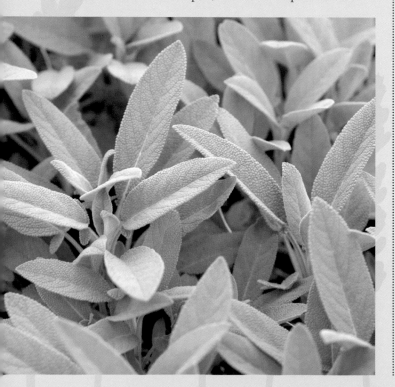

Santalum album – Santalaceae

Sandalwood

Sandalwood is an evergreen tree that is semi-parasitic. I went to India in the 1980s to learn its story and was fascinated to discover its dependence on other trees – for seven years it seeks nourishment from its neighbours' roots, eventually causing their death! It grows well around the areas of Mysore and Madras in India, although other varieties grow in Australasia and the Pacific Islands.

Benefits

* Anti-ageing
* Helps with eczema
* Smoothes wrinkles
* Helps thread veins, skin eruptions
* Good for the eyes
* Helps with cystitis and other bladder infections
* Eases bloating before periods
* Aphrodisiac
* Good for the pulmonary and respiratory systems
* Bactericide
* Used in perfume

Sandalwood was mentioned in ancient Sanskrit texts as having magical properties and was used regularly as a purifier for the soul and mind. It was used as incense in religious ceremonies (its bark was burnt to honour the gods) and also as a treatment for venereal disease. Ancient Egyptians used it in medicine and its wood was carved into sacred objects and boxes. It was also made into a healing balm and was said to be a wonderful aid to communication and overcoming shyness.

Today the role of sandalwood is one of rejuvenation and healing, and it is used for its anti-ageing properties. When used on skin, it becomes more soft and supple. It works on wrinkles and fine lines too!

The tree is sacred in India and has government protection – the trees have to be declared and authorization given before the grower is allowed to distil the essential oil. The tree needs to be at least 40 or 50 years old before it is mature enough for the oil to be obtained (this is found in both the roots and the centre of the trunk). It is a beautiful brown colour and has a woody, resinous, fruity aroma. In the 1970s, India produced over 200 tonnes a year. That figure has since markedly decreased because the trees are now so scarce.

It is used extensively in Ayurvedic medicine especially in treating cases of strong anxiety and depression and always accompanies a spiritual life as a meditation aid.

Today the role of sandalwood is one of rejuvenation and healing, and is used for its anti-ageing properties. When used on skin, it becomes more soft and supple. It works on wrinkles and fine lines too!

Lots of work has been carried out by the central pharmacy in France proving its bactericide properties, especially in the treatment of urinary infections such as cystitis and those caused by labour and childbirth. It has been prescribed both internally and externally to treat swellings due to bladder infections.

Sandalwood is used a great deal in perfume as it has a wonderful rich, balsamic aroma and is a natural fixative. It is used regularly in the Indian cosmetics industry.

Dangers

Essential oil of sandalwood is very often falsified because of its high cost. Be careful when buying oils as some may be adulterated with sesame or linseed oils, or even paraffin.

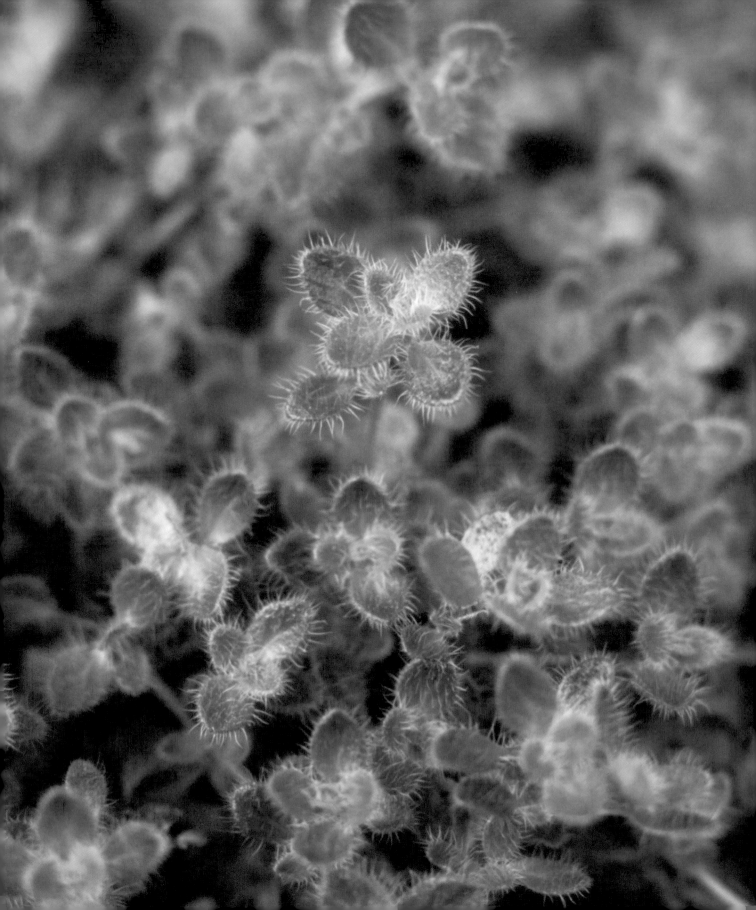

Thymus spp. – Labiatae

Thyme

Thyme grows in particular abundance in the Mediterranean countries but it can also be found all over the world.

Benefits

※ Helps with skin problems, dermatitis, acne
※ Helps ward off colds, flu, viruses
※ Treats dandruff
※ Eases rheumatic pain, lumbago, muscular pain, sciatica
※ Helps with depression
※ Relieves tiredness
※ Rejuvenating properties

Over 300 species of this hardy perennial plant have been recorded. The most common varieties of thyme include *T. citriodorus*, which has a lemony scent and *T. vulgaris*, the culinary thyme. It has dark green leaves, sometimes with a silver tone, and tiny tubular flowers that can vary in colour from bluish-pink to white and dark crimson depending on the species.

The origin of the word thyme is in the Greek *thumos*, or smell, as the plant is so aromatic. An old civilization, the Sumerians, were said to have used it as long ago as 3500 BC, while the Ancient Egyptians called it *tham* and used it in embalming.

Hippocrates included it in his 400 remedies, using it in infusions, as a cooking ingredient mixed with wine and applied externally. It was also regularly used in rituals and religious ceremonies as part of the offerings made to gods. Later the Romans found it useful for treating epilepsy and as a carminative, and soldiers bathed in thyme before a battle as a way of masking fear. Pliny added it to vinegar to cure headaches and migraines. It was also used as an antidote to snakebites and bunches were burnt outside homes to keep reptiles at bay. St Hildegarde prescribed thyme for leprosy and it has been strewn on floors as an anti-bacterial.

It has been claimed that thyme acts as an antioxidant fighting against free radicals to preserve human tissue. It helps soothe dermatitis and skin problems, and makes a good astringent to combat acne. Add it to a lotion for use before shampooing to get rid of dandruff. On its own in a tea, I have found it helpful for depression, tiredness and stress but it can also increase the therapeutic value of other oils (for example rose and bois de rose) when added to them. It is wonderful in the treatment of lumbago, rheumatic conditions, muscular pain and as a flu/virus preventative. The thymol content means the oil is good for reducing swellings. Doctors Leclerc and Bélaiche recommend a thyme tisane after a meal to help with the symptoms of old age.

Dangers

Be sure to buy 100% organic oil from a good supplier as essential oil of thyme is often adulterated.

It has been claimed that thyme acts as an antioxidant fighting against free radicals to preserve human tissue. It helps soothe dermatitis and skin problems, and makes a good astringent to combat acne.

Styrax benzoin – Styraceae

Benzoin

Originating in Laos and Vietnam, the *Styrax benzoin* tree now also grows in Malaysia, Java, Borneo and Sumatra, where it is highly cultivated.

Benefits

* Helps eczema, psoriasis
* Reduces the appearance of age spots on hands
* Treats wounds, burns
* Helps chest infections
* Treats colds and flu

The gum resin benzoin comes from the *Styrax benzoin* tree. The *Styrax benzoin* tree reaches about 20m (65ft) in height. Ancient Egyptian papyri stated that benzoin got to Egypt via the Red Sea. In old texts, benzoin is also called oil of ben, benjoin and benjamin. In Arabic it is called *luban-jawi* or 'incense from Sumatra'.

Benzoin is a sweet-smelling oleo resin that is obtained by a process using a solvent, which is removed later on with an alcohol. It has a wonderful, heavy, lingering aroma and must have given the perfume of the Ancients a warm and pleasant note.

Mixed and pounded together with frankincense and myrrh, and sometimes juniper, galbanum, labdenum and cypress, benzoin was used in rituals to venerate the gods (especially Râ, the sun god). The Ancient Greeks called it 'Silphion' and the Romans 'Laserpitium'. Both loved the powdered resin for its powerful fixative qualities, and it became an essential ingredient of their perfumes.

In Chinese medicine benzoin is considered yang (hot and related to the sun). It energizes, uplifts and promotes a special level of consciousness for meditation.

In England a tincture of benzoin compound (Friar's balsam) was used to treat external ulcers and as an inhalant for pulmonary disorders. Queen Elizabeth I wore benzoin-scented gloves in bed to help keep her hands pale and perfumed. During her reign, people used it to scent corsets, girdles and necklaces. Small bowls of powdered benzoin were placed near a fire or added to hot coals to perfume a room. Fragrances using benzoin were used to impregnate cloths, coat hangers, notepaper and wigs, a practice that came from France, Portugal and Spain.

During the reign of Louis XIV in France the use of heavy perfumes was in vogue and balsamic-smelling benzoin was often added as a fixative. Just like in England, it was used to perfume wigs, fine shirts and laced clothes. Censers were used to release the powerful aromas of vanilla and chocolate.

The French referred to benzoin as '*beaume pulmonaire*' (pulmonary balm) and classified it as an anti-spasmodic and as a tonic for many skin infections and eruptions. Sweets for colds and flu, '*pastilles de serail*', are based on benzoin and remedies using the resin help asthma and coughs.

Physician and chemist Dr Nicolas Lemery used benzoin for minor skin injuries and burns and mixed it into a pommade. He also found it useful in the treatment of skin complaints such as psoriasis, eczema, couperose and acne.

I love it added to perfume as it gives a warmth and strength to other fragrances, acting as an amplifier.

The principal constituents are approx 70–80% resin and 20–25% cinnamic acid, which are good for pulmonary problems as well as having antiseptic properties. The particular scent comes from the small quantities of vanillin and benzoic acid present.

Dangers

Be sure to do a skin test first as benzoin can cause allergic reactions in some people.

Vetiveria zizanioides/Andropogon muricatus – Gramineae

Vetiver

Vetiver essential oil is cultivated in tropical and sub-tropical climates such as the Seychelles, Java, India, China and Japan. However the oil that comes from the island of Réunion is considered the best.

Benefits

* Helps with skin problems
* Good for stress and tension
* Strengthens immune system
* Helps anaemia and blood loss
* Alleviates insomnia
* Used in perfume
* Good insect repellant

Vetiver oil comes from vetiver grass, part of the *Gramineae* family, which also includes wheat and rice. The aromatic substances accumulate in the roots of the grass – these are then distilled. The grasses are considered as sacred forms of nourishment and as gifts from the gods.

The grass grows in swamps and has strong, resistant roots that can survive storms and drought. In India people use it to ward off mosquitoes by making fans with the roots. They hang these in cupboards and over windows (they also exude a wonderful smell).

The aroma of vetiver is similar to that of musk with a note of sandalwood. It is earthy and woody and very uplifting. In India it is called the essential oil of tranquillity and it is given the name of 'khas-khas' or 'khus-khus'. The oil is dark brown in colour and the principal constituent is the alcohol, vetiverol. The aroma is difficult to reproduce synthetically, since it is so agreeable and full

Research has shown that vetiver encourages the production of red blood cells and has been given in cases of anaemia and prescribed to patients who have lost a lot of blood after operations.

of character. It is said to help control strong emotions.

Vetiver was introduced to me by Marguerite Maury who used it to strengthen the immune system, as a sedative and to help blood circulation. Research by Dr Valnet has shown that vetiver encourages the production of red blood cells and has been given in cases of anaemia and prescribed to patients who have lost a lot of blood after operations.

Fragile capillaries on the face and legs can benefit from an external application of vetiver as it helps to strengthen them. It also helps to combat greasy skin, nervous facial tension, muscular tension and insomnia. In times of stress, the essential oil can help bring back a clear mental state and aid relaxation.

Vetiver can also be added to cupboards and drawers to protect cashmere and woollen items from moths. Just add a few drops to blotting paper and place as necessary. It smells much better than moth balls!

Dangers

Vetiver is expensive to produce and is therefore sometimes adulterated. The resulting 'fake' oil can be harmful to the skin so its usage is now restricted. Make sure you buy pure vetiver oil from a good source.

Viola odorata – Violaceae

Violet leaves

Violet oil is cultivated in France and Europe.

Benefits
* Strengthens capillaries and veins
* Helps ease coughs
* Used in perfume

Violets are the symbol of the great city of Athens. In Ancient Greece they made crowns of violets to protect from drunkenness! It is said that Venus fell in love with Vulcan when he came to her wearing a crown of violets. They are given at funerals as a memorial and as a 'bridge' to the dead. Ancient poets Homer and Virgil made references to violets and described how they were used in tisanes to moderate anger in patients.

In the time of Louis XIV in France, it was the fashion to add violets to salads as they were said to help constipation. Violets were made into syrups for bad coughs. Folklore states that an aphrodisiac is produced when violets and lavender are taken together! Violets are also said to bring the mentally disturbed to their senses.

In aromatherapy, concrete (see page 6) violet is rarely used except when added to some body oils as a perfume. The leaves give an interesting leafy scent when added to perfume compositions and I love their base notes. The absolute extract is a very deep dark green and contains the constituent viola quercitine, which gives it its earthy, leafy scent.

Many years ago, when violet flower essential oil could still be found Marguerite Maury used it for a weak heart and to strengthen capillaries and veins. She prescribed violet essential oil to asthmatics to sniff during an attack and recommended taking a violet syrup for a bad cough.

Place a violet flower at the bottom of a glass of champagne, and wait for a few minutes for the sugary matter and the aroma to disperse through the drink. The violet will perfume the champagne and will give it a slightly nutty taste – great for parties!

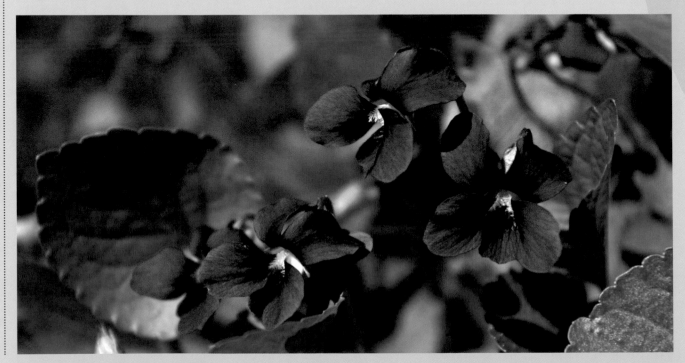

Zingiber officinalis – Zingiberaceae

Ginger

Ginger is native to Asia. It is also grown in South America and the West Indies. The best-quality oil comes from the West Indies.

Benefits

* Rejuvenating, repairing, restoring
* Stimulant: helps with fatigue and physical exhaustion
* Eases muscle tension
* Stomachic
* Tonic for digestion
* Decongestant: helps sinus problems; colds
* Aphrodisiac (especially for men)

Ginger is a tropical herbaceous plant that grows to just under 1m (3ft) in height and has spiky leaves that are similar in appearance to reeds. I love its orchid-like flowers as they have a wonderful aromatic fragrance.

Ginger was one of the first spices to reach Europe from Asia. The Spanish in America loved it for its therapeutic properties and cultivated it with great enthusiasm. The Spanish conquistadors introduced it to the West Indies.

The Ancient Egyptians revered ginger for its immune-boosting qualities. The Romans used ginger in their treatment of advanced cataracts – a ginger preparation was made up and applied to the eyes twice a day. Later, St Hildegarde swore by it for eye infections and diseases. She also mentioned its aphrodisiac qualities and claimed it was useful for stimulating the vigour of older men! In Senegal, women make a belt out of ginger roots and present it to their husbands or boyfriends in order to awaken their sexual desire.

It is the perfect root for the winter months – it can

In Senegal, women make a belt out of ginger roots and present it to their husbands or boyfriends in order to awaken their sexual desire.

be ground and added to dishes, crystallized in sugar or pickled. Ginger will always spice up your cooking.

Approx 300kg (660lb) of dried ginger roots are needed to produce 30kg (66lb) of essential oil. It is pale yellow in colour with a strong and penetrating, spicy, hot smell. The principal constituents are sesquiterpenes (camphrene, d-phellandrene and zingiberene), which are warming, decongestic and good for the stomach.

Dangers

Essential oil of ginger can be adulterated with other harmful oils so take care when purchasing. The adulterated oil will be a brownish yellow. Never use neat oil on the skin and never add it to your bath – you could end up with a nasty rash, blisters and a sore bottom!

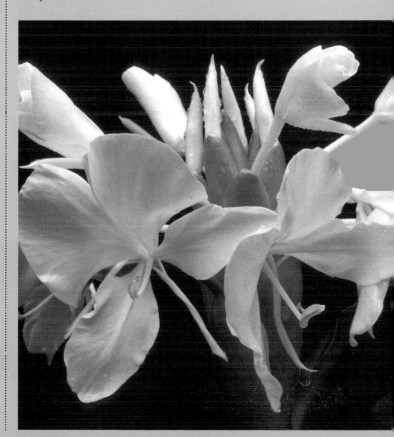

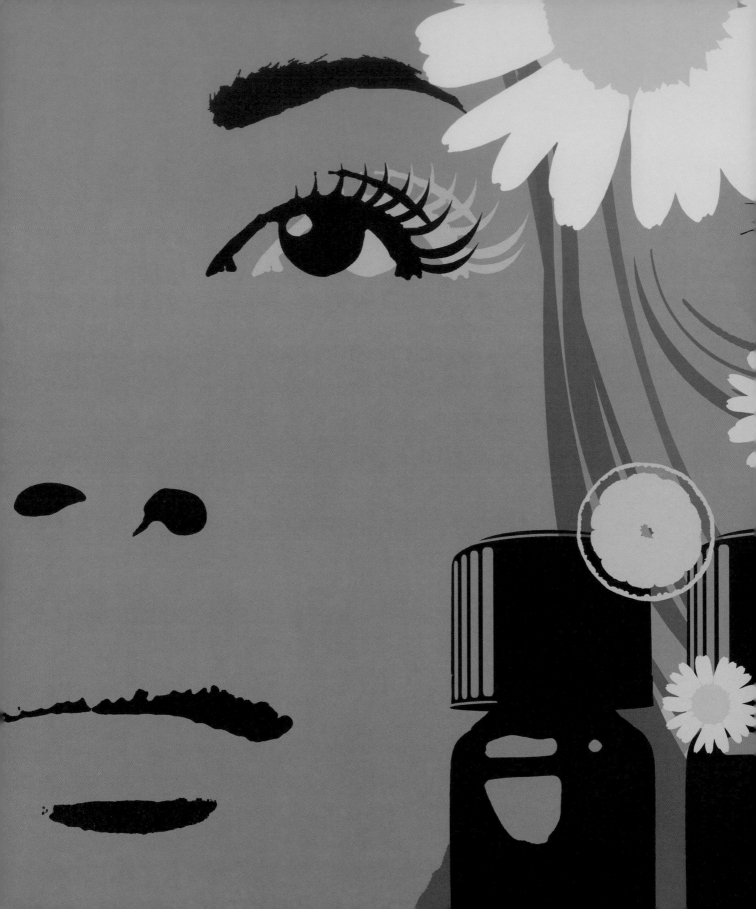

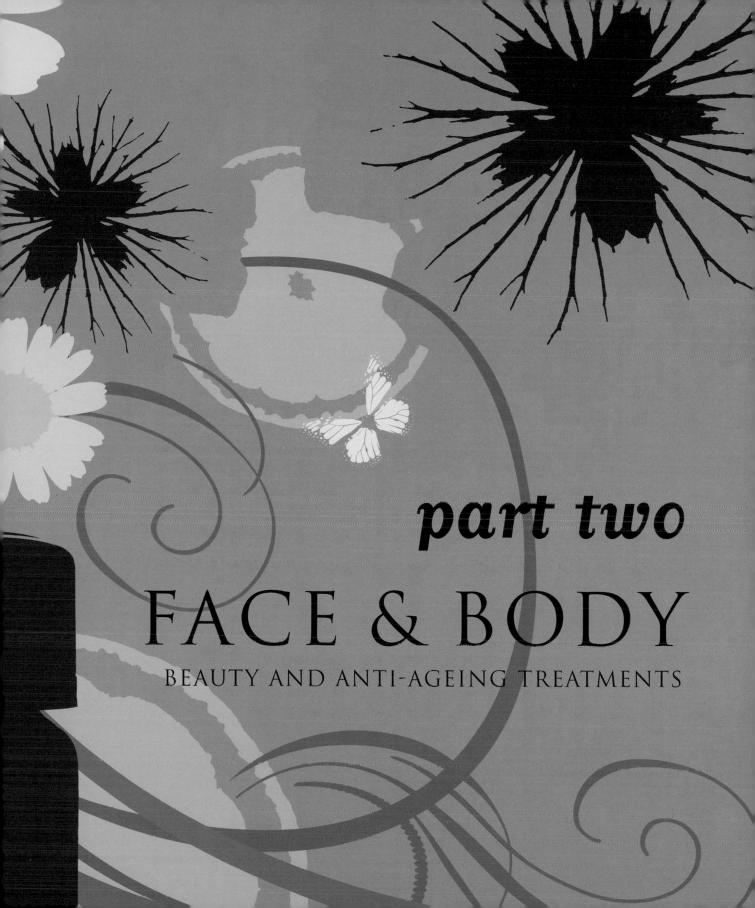

part two

FACE & BODY

BEAUTY AND ANTI-AGEING TREATMENTS

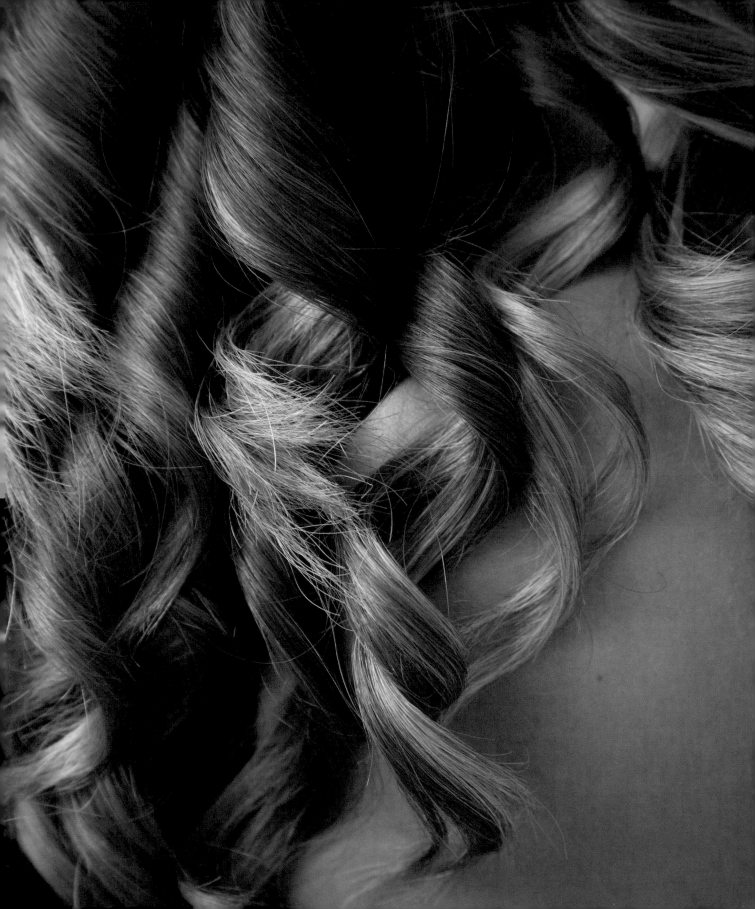

Hair and scalp care

Essential oils are extremely helpful in hair care as they influence the sebaceous glands, normalizing their functions. They benefit all hair types, and leave it smelling good too.

So much money is spent every day on our hair – on conditioning, perming, shampooing, colouring, setting, cutting – and to most women it is their most important asset. Well conditioned hair can literally knock years off your appearance. New products, giving ample promises, come on to the market regularly. They are extensively advertised and some are celebrity endorsed, so we feel we need to have them. Most of the time we don't.

The scalp is one of the five principal sensory organs and is therefore subject to some of the same general problems that beset the skin. I am always amazed that the scalp doesn't react more severely to the strong shampoos and conditioners we use, perms, blow-drying, hair extensions and chemical hair colours (recently twenty-two toxic substances, found in hair dyes, sprays and salon shampoos, were banned because they were found to be irritants to the skin). Just think of what these strong chemicals do to the environment. Our rivers and water supplies are becoming more and more polluted. Why not save money and go for a more natural approach?

There are approximately 100,000 hairs on our heads, each made of a strong stretchable protein material called keratin. The hair itself is dead but, even so, its condition still depends on a good diet, and smoking is one of the most common causes of dull and damaged hair! A period of ill health, shock (I remember when I was eleven, my best friend had such a shock that her hair turned white within a week!), stress or poor nutrition (anorexia for example) can all affect the hair's appearance. Beauty,

A diet rich in minerals helps the condition of the scalp and citrus fruits can add to the shine of the hair.

strength and shine, even the hair itself, will be lost. These symptoms can be particularly apparent during times of emotional upheaval – menopausal women can experience thinning hair and adolescents can suffer from overactive sebaceous glands that result in spots, greasy hair, itchy scalp and dandruff.

People worry about going grey and for a young face it can be a difficult colour to carry off. People cover it because they see it as a sign of ageing but dyeing your hair can also damage it. Grey hair can be elegant and distinguished and by continually dyeing it we are just putting more money into the manufacturers' pockets.

Preventing hair problems with a good diet is essential, so make sure you have plenty of vitamin B (pantothenate or panthothenic acid, found in vitamin B complex, is especially good for stress-related hair problems) – nuts, wheatgerm and fish oils are all good sources. A diet rich in minerals helps the condition of the scalp and citrus fruits can add to the shine of the hair.

Essential oils to use for normal hair:
Lemon, geranium, cedarwood, bois de rose, carrot and lavender

Essential oils to use for dry hair:
Lavender, sandalwood and myrrh

Essential oils to use for grey hair:
Cade, rosemary and sage

Essential oils to use for greasy hair:
Rosemary, tea tree, thyme, eucalyptus, melissa, lavender, geranium and cedarwood

Essential oils to use for weak/damaged hair:
Chamomile, calendula, cypress, bergamot, melissa, patchouli, basil and sandalwood

Making your own shampoos and conditioners

Always use a natural, clear, fragrance-free shampoo as a base. Health food shops usually stock a good range. Mix the appropriate essential oil with it, shaking well. It is important to leave the bottle to 'settle' for at least ten days in order for it to work properly. It should then last for about two to three months.

Wash your hair two to three times a week, shampooing only once. If you need to wash it more frequently, dilute the preparation with water. Use your fingertips to gently massage the scalp and stimulate the hair follicles. Hair should be conditioned once or twice a month.

Shampoo for normal hair

100ml bottle of shampoo (as above)
2 drops essential oil of cedarwood
4 drops essential oil of bois de rose
1 drop essential oil of lemon

Shake well, leave for ten days before use. ❧

Shampoo for greasy hair

100ml bottle of shampoo (as above)
2 drops essential oil of melissa
5 drops essential oil of lavender
5 drops essential oil of geranium
1 drop essential oil of cedarwood

Shake well, leave for ten days before use. ❧

Shampoo for dry/damaged hair

100ml bottle of shampoo (as above)
5 drops essential oil of cypress
2 drops essential oil of bergamot
4 drops essential oil of melissa
2 capsules wheatgerm oil

Shake well, leave for ten days before use. ❧

Shampoo and conditioner (all in one) for dry and damaged hair

2 egg yolks (egg yolks are great emulsifiers and wonderful for softening and conditioning the hair)
15ml (1 tablespoon) of vodka
1 drop essential oil of lemon
1 drop essential oil of tea tree

Mix up in a bowl. Shampoo your hair with the mixture, cover with a shower cap. Leave on for five to ten minutes, then rinse. Important – make sure you rinse out with tepid/lukewarm water otherwise you may find you have an omelette on the top of your head!

Finish with a cold rinse to bring shine to the hair. ❧

Conditioner for dry hair with split ends

When there aren't enough sebum secretions being released, the hair becomes more fragile and starts to break. Bleaching, blow-drying and colouring exacerbate the condition. When on holiday it is a good idea to protect your hair from the sun and avoid seawater and chlorine.

3–4 capsules lecithin, strong strength (see page 73)
5ml (1 teaspoon) sesame oil
5ml (1 teaspoon) castor oil
5ml (1 teaspoon) grapeseed oil
3ml (1/2 teaspoon) argan oil
1 capsule wheatgerm oil
1 capsule evening primrose oil
1 teaspoon cocoa butter
2 drops essential oil of myrrh
2 drops essential oil of sandalwood

In a bain-marie, mix the lecithin with the sesame, castor, grapeseed, argan, wheatgerm and evening primrose oils. Stir in the cocoa butter until softened. Remove from the heat and add the essential oil of myrrh and sandalwood. Apply to damp hair massaging it into the scalp and ends. Leave on for ten to fifteen minutes. Shampoo off and rinse with cold water. For a last rinse, mix one tablespoon cider vinegar and either a squeeze of lemon juice if you have blonde hair or two drops essential oil of clary sage or rosemary if you have dark hair, in a glass of boiled, bottled water. ❧

❧ *Many labels on shampoo bottles don't always list all the ingredients and some can be very strong. I always recommend that you shampoo your hair only once – it isn't that dirty! People with greasy hair should dilute the shampoo as well; this will avoid irritation, dandruff and keep it in good condition.*

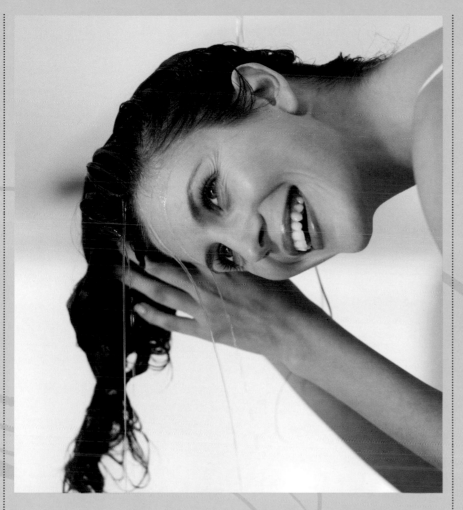

tablespoon cider vinegar and two drops essential oil of geranium in a glass of boiled, bottled water. ❧

Conditioner for greasy hair

I believe that people who have greasy hair shouldn't use conditioners. Their hair is oily already and the oil is a natural conditioner anyway. The best thing to do is shampoo and finish with a last rinse for your hair colour.

Volumizing scalp rub

This will give the hair lots of volume and make it really shiny!

20ml (2 dessert spoons) grapeseed oil
1 capsule wheatgerm oil
1 capsule evening primrose oil
20 drops essential oil of lavender
5 drops essential oil of ylang-ylang

Twice a week, before shampooing, rub your scalp vigorously with this oil. Leave on for a few minutes before shampooing it out. ❧

Dry shampoo for all hair types

This is a great way to instantly freshen the hair between shampoos.

1 small cup of fragrance-free talcum powder
4 drops either essential oil of jasmine or rosemary (or 2 of each)

Add the essential oils to the talcum powder. Mix together then leave overnight. Transfer to a shaker and shake over your hair, rubbing the scalp. Leave on for a few moments before brushing out. ❧

Conditioner for normal hair

Conditioner for normal hair must be rich in proteins and my favourite is lecithin – a protein made from soya. You can buy it from health food shops in granules or capsules. I prefer to use the capsules because you can sometimes get lumps with the granules. Lecithin combined with essential oils will nourish, moisturize and protect your hair, making it healthier and shinier.

2 capsules of lecithin, strong strength
10ml (1 dessert spoon) soya oil
1 capsule wheatgerm oil
1 teaspoon cocoa butter
4 drops essential oil of geranium
2 drops essential oil of lavender

In a bain-marie, mix the lecithin with the soya and wheatgerm oils, and the cocoa butter. Stir with a wooden spoon until melted. Remove from the heat and add the geranium and lavender. Apply to damp hair, massaging it into the scalp and ends. Leave on for ten to fifteen minutes. Shampoo off and rinse with cold water. For a last rinse, mix one

Colouring and styling hair

The Ancient Egyptians, Greeks and Romans all utilized natural dyes for their hair to achieve a more natural (and I think better) result than we see nowadays.

Records tell us that approximately four thousand years ago henna was used by Egyptian women to dye their hair and wigs. They mixed it with essential oils to make it smell nice.

Ancient Greeks bleached their hair with saffron while the Romans favoured walnut shells to give their hair a reddish tint.

Setting lotions

Dark hair

50ml lager (any kind will do)
50ml water
*1 drop either essential oil of clary
    sage or rosemary*
100ml spray bottle

Pour into the bottle and use in place of hairspray. Apply to damp hair and style as usual.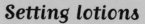

Blonde hair

Lemon juice is excellent for blonde hair, bringing both highlights and shine. I have been using it as a setting lotion since my youth and have never needed any other hairspray. This recipe will also give volume to fine hair and restore lustre.

Juice of one lemon
100ml water
1 drop essential oil of ylang-ylang
100ml spray bottle

Mix well in a bowl then pour into a spray bottle. Use to spray hair after shampooing and before styling.

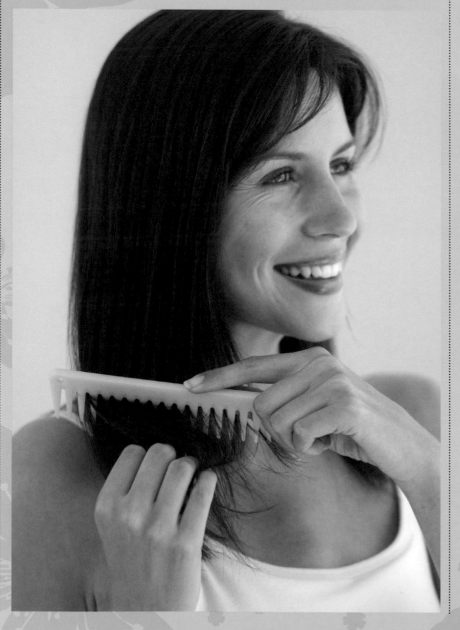

Colouring treatments

Cade hair oil for greying hair

This will help prevent grey hair from turning white.

20ml (2 dessert spoons) grapeseed oil
1 capsule wheatgerm oil
1 capsule evening primrose oil
6 drops essential oil of cade

First massage the scalp with your fingers to warm it up. Apply the oil and massage into the scalp, pressing firmly with your fingertips. Leave on for a couple of hours then wash with a gentle shampoo: add ten drops of essential oil of cade to 150ml natural fragrance-free shampoo. Mix and wash hair once. Follow by a cold rinse. Use two or three times a month. ❧

Cade lotion for greying hair

Most of us think of old age when we see grey hair and instantly reach for the hair dye. But instead of choosing a chemical-laden solution, why not try something more natural? Nowadays there are many natural ways to cover grey, with lots of salons catering for the demand, but it is just as easy to make your own at home.

30ml (2 tablespoons) soya oil
15ml (1 tablespoon) grapeseed oil
1 capsule wheatgerm oil
6 drops essential oil of cade

Mix together before massaging into hair and scalp, leave on five to ten minutes. Shampoo off. (Make your own shampoo for this – add twelve drops of essential oil of cade to a 150ml bottle natural, fragrance-free shampoo.) Use two or three times a month. ❧

Chamomile hair tonic for blonde hair

Chamomile helps lighten blonde hair, as it is a natural bleach.

12 flower heads of chamomile or
  5 chamomile tea bags
600ml (1 pint) boiling water
2 drops essential oil of chamomile
10ml (1 dessert spoon) of vodka
1 large bottle

Add the flower heads or the tea bags to a teapot and cover with 600ml (1 pint) of boiling water. Leave to steep and infuse for several hours. Strain. Add the vodka (it acts as a preservative) and the chamomile essential oil. Transfer to a bottle. You can use this tonic to massage the scalp between shampoos or added to the last rinse after shampooing. This quantity should make enough for approximately ten applications and should keep for two to three months. ❧

Rosemary hair tonic for dark hair

Rosemary helps condition dark hair and maintains the colour.

6 sprigs of fresh rosemary
600ml (1 pint) boiling water
10ml (1 dessert spoon) of dark rum
2 drops essential oil of rosemary
1 large bottle

Add the rosemary sprigs to a teapot and cover with 600ml (1 pint) of boiling water. Leave to steep and infuse for several hours. Strain, then add the rum and essential oil of rosemary. Transfer to a bottle and leave to rest in the dark for a week. Use as a tonic lotion to massage the hair and scalp between shampoos, or added to the last rinse after shampooing. ❧

Sage hair tonic for greying hair

Sage is wonderful for 'salt and pepper' hair as it slightly darkens it, keeping the colour.

5 sage leaves
500ml water

In a small saucepan, bring the sage leaves and the water to the boil. Remove and let cool, infusing for half-an-hour. Strain. Use as a final rinse after shampooing. ❧

Lacklustre hair

Revitalizing dull hair

A few nights without sleep makes your hair dull, fragile and even encourages hair-loss! Brushing is a great way to put the life back in to it, especially when combined with a hair tonic (see below). Make sure you have a good bristle brush, it'll be like a scalp massage and you will see the results in a short time.

Hair tonic

Pour a couple of drops of either essential oil of rosemary or ylang-ylang on the palm of your hand and rub into your hair and scalp. Put your head down and brush your hair vigorously, section by section, finishing at the front. ❧

Hair problems

Dandruff

Most people suffer from the common problem of dandruff at some point in their lives. Skin cells on the scalp are continuously renewing themselves, the dead ones falling as dandruff. Another cause is *pityriasis capitis* or scaly head, which makes the head very itchy and sometimes makes the scalp smelly. It is important to treat both these problems. It is better to let your hair dry naturally as hairdryers dry out the scalp; if you must use one make sure it is set to a cool temperature and don't hold it too close to the scalp. Avoid using hairsprays and mousses as these will leave residues and accentuate the condition. Humidity is also important so drink plenty of water and spray water in the air where you work; alternatively, place a bowl of hot water near your desk.

Dandruff treatment

Make up this shampoo at least ten days before using to allow the mixture to settle.

*5 drops essential oil of rosemary, tea
   tree, lavender or myrrh*
1–2 capsules wheatgerm oil
1 capsule evening primrose oil

Mix well in a bowl then massage into your scalp gently. Leave on for thirty minutes before washing with the following shampoo:

*100ml natural, clear, fragrance-free
   shampoo (organic ingredients if
   possible)*
7 drops essential oil of tea tree
1 drop essential oil of myrrh
3 drops essential oil of cedarwood

It is important to wash your hair gently, massaging your scalp for a few minutes. Rinse your hair with warm, not hot, water, making sure all traces of shampoo have disappeared. Finish with a cold-water rinse, taking your time. Continue treatment for a month or until the condition has improved. (Use up to three times a week.) ❧

Hair lotion for dandruff and greasy hair

This is a wonderful lotion to use between shampoos and you don't need to rinse it out.

*2 sprigs fresh rosemary or 4
   chamomile flower heads (if you
   can't find them a chamomile tea
   bag will suffice)*
10ml (1 dessert spoon) cider vinegar
5 drops essential oil of tea tree
100ml bottle

> ❧ *To avoid bacterial infections – don't scratch your itchy scalp. The condition could worsen and you might break the skin.*

Add your chosen herb to 600ml (1 pint) of water. Boil for two minutes then remove from the heat and cover. Leave to infuse for twenty-five minutes before letting cool and transferring enough to nearly fill a 100ml bottle. Add the cider vinegar and tea tree oil when the mixture has cooled down. Rub gently into your scalp at night, massaging it in with the fingertips. This will keep for two to three weeks. ❧

Weak hair

Hair can become weak and lifeless after a long illness or period of ill health. This hair strengthening oil can be very useful.

5ml (1 teaspoon) flax oil
5ml (1 teaspoon) castor oil
2 drops essential oil of patchouli

Warm the oils slightly using a bain-marie. Remove from the heat. Add the patchouli and mix. Massage the hair with the preparation, covering with a shower cap and a warm towel. Leave for at least half-an-hour. Rinse off using a clear, fragrance-free shampoo with two drops of essential oil of patchouli added. Use two to three times a month. ❧

Hair extensions, blow-drying and diet can all affect our hair, but basil is a great healer. It strengthens the hair by providing it with nutrients, enabling the follicle to become more productive. It also stimulates the blood flow and increases circulation to the scalp. Add a drop of essential oil of basil to 1 litre of cold water (preferably filtered or mineral water). Shake well and use in place of the final rinse after shampooing.

Alopecia

Hair-loss of any type can be devastating. It can be caused by a number of different factors. Cancer treatments such as radiotherapy and chemotherapy are two of the most common but hormone imbalances and stress can also cause hair-loss. Sometimes women experience the condition during pregnancy or menopause.

Ylang-ylang hair-loss remedy

Ylang-ylang has long been used in hair treatments (the essential oil was once used in a nineteenth-century hair oil called Macassar). Before applying the oil, tip your head forwards and brush your hair until your scalp feels warm.

6 drops essential oil of ylang-ylang
1 capsule borage oil
1 capsule evening primrose oil
50ml bottle

Mix the oils and shake well. Massage the oil into your scalp one hour before shampooing. Use two to three times a month. You can also add a few drops of this oil to a mild shampoo. Shake the bottle and use in combination with the scalp oil. ஃ

Chamomile for hair-loss

If hair is thinning chamomile can help.

15 drops essential oil of chamomile
2 capsules wheatgerm oil
2 drops essential oil of sage or
*   clary sage*

Mix in a bowl. Twice a week, an hour before shampooing, massage your scalp with this oil. ஃ

Nutmeg scalp-rub for hair-loss

50ml water
50ml cider vinegar
½ grated nutmeg
10 drops essential oil of rosemary
1 teaspoon Manuka honey
100ml bottle

Pour the water, vinegar and nutmeg into a small saucepan and bring to the boil. Take off the heat and leave to infuse for half-an-hour. When cool, add the rosemary and honey. Use this preparation to massage the scalp twice a day for a few weeks. It's not greasy so you don't have to rinse it out. It will keep for about a month. Use in tandem with a natural shampoo containing ten drops of essential oil of nutmeg and three drops of cedarwood. ஃ

Split ends

Linseed poultice for split ends

5 tablespoons linseeds, crushed
5ml (1 teaspoon) flax oil
Boiling water
2 drops either essential oil of basil
*   or geranium*
Gauze

Crush the linseeds in a blender. Transfer to a small bowl and add the flax oil. Slowly add some boiling water – you want a paste-like consistency. Add the essential oil. Cut a gauze square big enough to cover your head and use a spatula to spread the paste over it. Cover with another piece of gauze and secure the corners by lightly rolling them. Wet your hair then roughly dry it (if you have long hair, pile it on top of your head). Place the gauze on top, covering with a shower cap and wrapping in a warm towel to help the oils penetrate the hair. Leave on for between half-an-hour and an hour. Remove the poultice and shampoo. Repeat once a month and be sure to have your hair cut regularly! ஃ

Pre-shampoo conditioner for split ends

Clary sage leaves are a great tonic. They condition and darken hair so are particularly good for those grey patches!

30ml (2 tablespoons) grapeseed oil
1 capsule wheatgerm oil
8 drops essential oil of clary sage
50ml bottle

Mix and pour into the bottle. When required, apply a little of the oil to the split ends. Wrap hair in a towel and leave for an hour. Will keep for about a month. Use a gentle shampoo to rinse out the oil, following with either lemon juice for blonde hair or cider vinegar for dark hair. ஃ

TREATING HEADACHE AND MIGRAINE

A simple headache could be caused by many different factors – colds and flu, stress, eyestrain or something more serious.

Many women suffer from headaches when they are pre-menstrual and often digestive problems can be a cause. Migraines, on the other hand, are severe, recurrent headaches and one of the most common disorders of the nervous system. They can be hereditary and they affect more women than men. You should always consult a doctor if a headache persists.

Headaches

Many things can bring on headaches so you need to treat different types with different oils. Put a drop of the particular oil on a tissue and inhale the fumes for a few moments, closing your eyes.

For headaches brought on by colds and flu, sinus problems and a blocked nose:

Geranium, cajuput, niaouli, pine, eucalyptus and tea tree.
Inhalation is especially good to clear catarrh, which can provoke headaches. Use on a tissue or add two oils, one drop of each, to a bowl of hot water. Cover your head with a towel and inhale for a few minutes.

For general headaches that come on for no apparent reason:

Geranium and chamomile.
Put a drop of each on a tissue and inhale, closing your eyes.

For headaches caused by stress or anxiety:

Petit grain, neroli and lavender.
Again put one drop of your chosen oil on a tissue and inhale.

For hangover headaches:

Black pepper, juniper and citrus oils, such as mandarin and orange.
Try relaxing in a bath with two to four drops of your chosen essential oil to pep you up.

Eyestrain

Cover your eyes with the palms of your hands for a few moments. Eye compresses would also be beneficial – try chamomile, rosemary or parsley (see page 11).

Migraines

Up to 5 per cent of the population suffer from migraines and they can be particularly common in energetic, stressed people. Triggers include certain foods, smells, wine and the contraceptive pill.

Essential oils that can help with migraines include:

Basil, chamomile, fennel, lemongrass, melissa, marjoram and oregano.

Basil oil for migraines

Basil is wonderfully effective for migraines so as soon as you feel the symptoms coming on, infuse a handful of fresh basil in hot water and drink. You can also add it to your food – omelettes, pasta, salad etc. or try this massage oil.

10ml (1 dessert spoon) grapeseed oil
1 capsule wheatgerm oil
3 drops essential oil of basil
50ml bottle

Mix ingredients together in the bottle and shake well. Massage the oil into the temples, around the sinus area and on the nape of the neck. Lie down in a quiet place with a damp towel on your forehead. Relax. This oil will keep for two to three months. (You can also place a drop of essential oil of basil into a bowl of hot water and place it beside you.)

Migraine compress

1 drop essential oil of Roman chamomile or bergamot
1 drop essential oil of petit grain

Add the essential oils to a bowl of hot water and plunge a flannel or a small towel into it. Squeeze out the excess water and place the towel on your forehead. Lie down with your feet elevated in a dark room away from noise.

RELIEVING STRESS AND ANXIETY

Essential oils have a valuable part to play in helping us to cope with stressful lives and the continuous demands of the twenty-first century.

They enable us to calm down and recharge our batteries – aromatherapy massages are especially good; try to have one at least once a week and you will reap the benefits in no time. Set aside a special treatment day and have a massage or an aromatherapeutic bath – do stretching exercises beforehand, since they will help you relax. Good essential oils for relaxation are: neroli, petit grain, orange and lavender.

Different types of stress

Stress in a normal state

Positive stress goes with excitement and positive things – enjoying what you are doing and doing it to the full. Your energy is stimulated by challenges and your body responds in such a way in order to cope with it.
Good stimulants for the nervous system are: *geranium, basil, rosemary and neroli.*

Use in a bath or vaporized in your room/near your work desk. You can also rub a drop on your sinuses, nape of neck, torso and lower back before you get into the shower.

Physical stress

Physical stress arises when you are at the limit of what you can achieve. Working for too long, driving long distances or hard exercise can all make demands on your energy.

Good oils for recuperation are: *thyme, peppermint, lavender, melissa and marjoram.*

Nervous stress

This is the feeling you experience during exams, if you have financial problems or are feeling overwhelmed.
Good oils for nervous stress are: *rose, neroli, orange, basil, sandalwood, patchouli.*

Emotional stress

This can be experienced during bereavement. Or you may feel it when you are going through a divorce.
Good oils for emotional stress are: *bois de rose, mandarin, neroli, rose, cedarwood, geranium, eucalyptus.*

Stress caused by the environment

This can result from exposure to too many pollutants at home or work, bad eating habits, taking drugs or not taking enough exercise.
Good oils for stress caused by the environment are: *cypress, pine, grapefruit, lemon and petit grain.*

Remedies for combating stress

The different types of stress can vary from good to bad. You can use the recommended essential oils above in the bath. Combine two or three,

adding no more than five or six drops of essential oil altogether.

Massage oil to relieve stress

10ml (1 dessert spoon) almond oil
1 capsule wheatgem oil
5–6 drops of your chosen essential oil

Mix together and massage into your torso, inhaling the fumes. Repeat several times throughout the day. You can also apply it to your wrists, solar plexus and back of the neck. ✄

Room spray

You can also vaporize the oils by filling a small spray bottle with mineral water and adding a few drops of essential oil. Spray it in the air around you and breathe in the fumes – it's an instant calmer. ✄

Meditative inhalation

Put a few drops of essential oil in a bowl of boiling water. Sit comfortably nearby, close your eyes, and inhale the fumes for a few minutes. ✄

Calming nerves

If you have to meet someone you don't particularly like or do something you know will make you nervous, apply a few drops of neat essential oil on your wrists and torso. The smell will act as a shield and make you feel more comfortable. Try clary sage, rose, geranium or neroli.

Facial skin care

I've always thought that human skin, the largest organ of the body, is one of the miracles of nature. For a person of a normal build, approximately 60kg (130lb), the skin will constitute approx 3kg (6½lb) of this weight. It is almost the thickness of a small coin, a little thicker on the palms of the hands, soles of the feet and at the nape of the neck. Our skin not only protects us from harmful bacteria but also helps eliminate toxins, waste and sweat. Oxygen and carbon dioxide pass in and out in a kind of respiration, akin to that which takes place in the lungs.

With all this in mind, essential oils are vital to the health and rejuvenation of the skin. Essential oils can safeguard the skin from foreign bodies, help with the elimination of waste and purify and oxygenate. It is now acknowledged that the volatile essential oil molecules can be diffused via the skin, reinforcing the fact that our biggest organ is also one of the most absorbent. Once the essential oils pass through the epidermis they seep into the small capillaries in the dermis and are then carried around the body in the blood. They also penetrate the lymph fluid that surrounds every cell in the body.

As it is in continual contact with the external environment, the skin plays an essential role in forming the first line of defence against bacteria and viruses found in the air around us. But thanks to their natural anti-bacterial and anti-viral properties, daily applications of essential oils keep it healthy, glowing and young. They also assist in the healing of cuts and wounds as they not only reduce the possibility of infection but also stimulate the regeneration of new skin cells – perfect for rejuvenation and keeping that youthful look!

Essential oils cleanse, purify, exfoliate and tone and are far cheaper than most beauty products on the market.

Look at your face; every face tells a story. Our faces reflect our emotions and each line and wrinkle represents something.

With a few drops you can achieve so much. All you have to do is follow the steps – cleanse, tone, moisturize, exfoliate and rejuvenate with masks and you will reap the benefits in no time.

Look at your face; every face tells a story. Our faces reflect our emotions and each line and wrinkle represents something, maybe a difficult time in our lives or even a liking for laughter. Expression lines can be beautiful, sexy and engaging – especially those that are caused by too much smiling! Sometimes, though, stress, nervousness, sadness and despair carve deeper lines into our faces, making us appear older and less attractive to others. We can hide our wrinkles with make-up but it won't hold for long and, if we haven't taken care, skin can become easily dehydrated, wrinkled and sensitive. Sometimes the sebaceous glands become overactive and the result is a greasy, shiny appearance. Pollution levels are a major cause, as many working environments have a lack of fresh air; sunlight has high levels of UV rays and many of us indulge in the odd cigarette and glass of wine. Bearing all this in mind, our skin, and our faces in particular, have a lot to put up with!

Normal skin

In my practice, I rarely see anyone with 'normal' skin. People with normal skin are lucky as they tend to have few problems but attention is needed to ensure the equilibrium is maintained and products have to be carefully selected. To tell if your skin is normal, close your eyes and place your fingertip on your forehead – it should feel slightly humid and damp. A good colour and glow are also important.

If your skin falls into the normal, balanced category make sure it stays that way by keeping away from harsh skin-care products and sticking to a good daily routine. Always use a moisturizer or spray your face with floral water. Drink plenty of water and eat a diet rich in fruit, vegetables and omega oils.

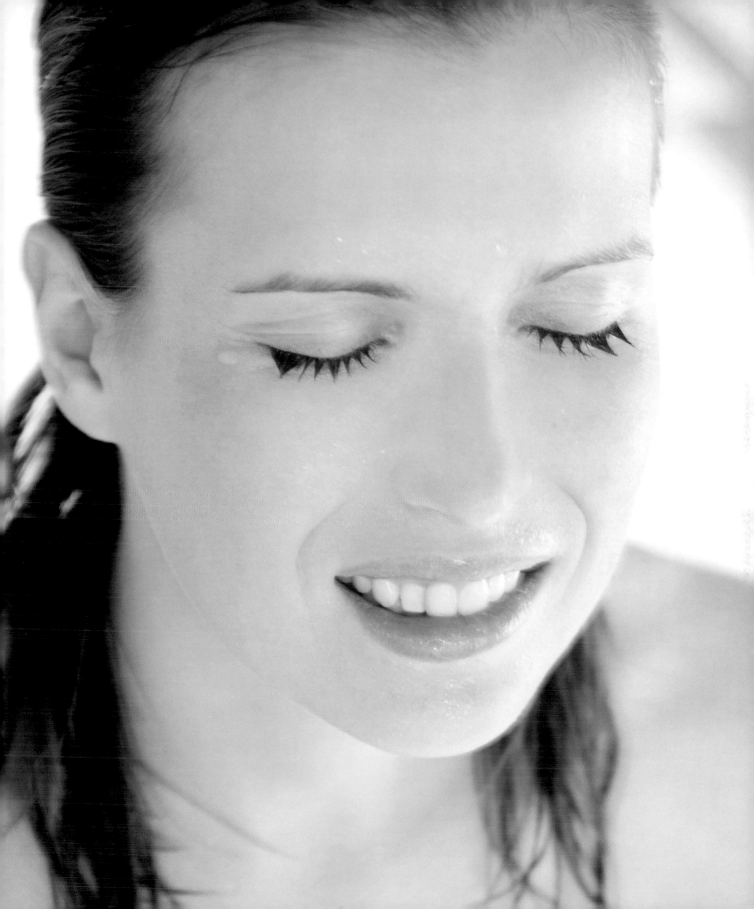

Combination skin

So many people have what is described as 'combination skin' and if you fall into this category you can mix and match all the recipes as you see fit, adjusting the preparations to get the best results. I have seen many clients with this skin type. Some have an oily area in the centre of the face with drier skin around the cheeks while others are the opposite – the cheeks are oily while the nose and forehead are drier. Try the treatments for normal skin, changing them slowly depending on how the different areas feel after a few weeks.

Mature skin

Every one of us dreads the appearance of wrinkles; they are a constant reminder of the passing years. After the birth of my son I remember my shock when I discovered a line on the side of my cheek, I was really upset.

As we get older cell division slows down and as a consequence the epidermis becomes thinner and the newly formed cells take longer to reach the surface so wrinkles are formed. But our attitude to life, our behaviour, beliefs, enthusiasm and the way we react to our environment can all determine the rate of ageing, so be happy!

Mature skins are so often extra-sensitive, having become more so over the years and this extra-sensitivity can result in premature ageing. I believe that some mature skin can regain its elasticity, collagen and firmness. Wrinkles can be smoothed, foreheads can appear tauter and lines on the neck can improve. This can be achieved by following a simple routine – use sensible products, wear little make-up and look after your health and diet. The right essential oils can dramatically improve things and skin will regain a more youthful look.

Mature skins tend to be very dehydrated so make sure you drink a lot of water, even better invest in a humidifier, as the air around us can be so drying. Herb teas are also wonderful but caffeine is not so good so try to limit your intake. Be especially careful in the summer months, as the sun, combined with the sudden change in temperature, and harsh sunscreens, can be very damaging.

Dry and sensitive skin

A dermatologist friend in Paris told me that in the last ten years there has been a marked increase in the number of people with dry and sensitive skin. She said that over 65% of people have experienced this condition and she has noted that skin seems to be ageing faster and faster. It is hard to understand why this happens when there are so many products on the market, all promising miracles. She said that people often have skin reactions to strong products, themselves causing premature ageing. We are all in effect acting as guinea-pigs for the new products – our skin flares up because they are strong, so then we use more of them. And all the while our skin becomes more sensitive. Beware of false promises and always check the products before buying; ask for a sample and wait at least two to four days to see if you have a reaction.

Dry skin results from an inability of the sebaceous glands to produce the correct quantity of oil needed to stop the skin losing moisture. As a consequence the skin feels taut and sometimes flaky. It loses its elasticity and suppleness and becomes prone to fine lines – the start of premature ageing. Some people also suffer from extra-sensitivity and red blotches. Illness and a diet deficient in vitamins A, C and E, minerals and essential fatty acids can all cause dry skin. Rapid weight loss and antibiotics also exacerbate the condition.

When your skin is on the dry side it has tiny cracks and can't do its job properly, so irritants get in. Make sure you drink enough water and place bowls of water around your home to increase the humidity in the air (add a few drops of either eucalyptus or lavender to the water). Facial sprays are great too and try not to wash your face with soap – it can be very drying.

Oily skin

During adolescence when the hormones are undergoing dramatic changes, it is quite common for the sebaceous glands to become overactive. The skin looks on the shiny side and often there are large pores on the nose, forehead and chin. Blackheads and spots, even acne, are common. Some people suffer more severely than others and a poor diet can be a factor. Stress can also cause problems –

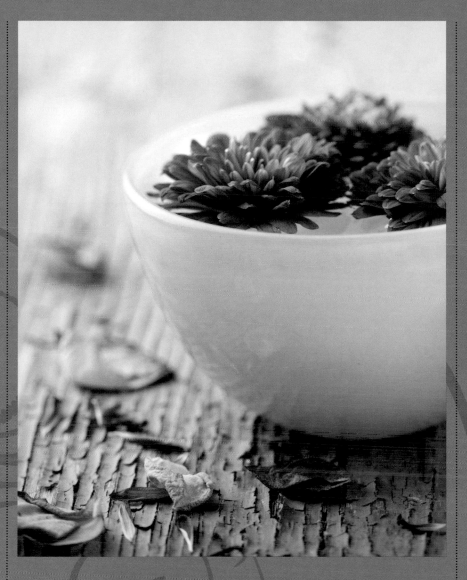

texture and circulation but you also need to eliminate the toxins so a good cleanser is the first step. Some cleansers on the market are too harsh; they interfere with the skin's natural function and can leave it feeling taut, tight and sensitive. It cannot do its job properly and will need continual attention. Some people even find they become extra-sensitive to water (if you have this problem, replace tap water with boiled or bottled water; you can even use chamomile tea). If you don't cleanse there is no point in putting any beauty products on your face, as nothing will be absorbed properly.

Taking time out to cleanse your face properly will improve the appearance of your skin but it is also important to try and relax the facial muscles before you begin the process. Smiling will automatically do this but essential oils can also help.

But first things first – before any beauty process you must make sure your hands are clean. Wash them thoroughly then rub them with a few drops of neat tea tree, petit grain, rosemary or lavender oil. Now you are ready to begin the cleansing procedure.

Start by relaxing your face. Fill your washbasin with hot water and add a drop of either lavender, petit grain, rose, neroli, basil or tea tree oil. Inhale the fumes for a few minutes before cleansing. (It is important to make sure that your hair is off your face – use a hair band or shower cap.)

more adrenalin is produced so the hormones are affected and things become unbalanced. Some oily skins can be extra-sensitive too so you have to take special care.

All these problems are easily remedied but you have to give things a chance to settle down. Too many harsh treatments can provoke even more oily secretions from skin that is desperate to replace what has been stripped away, setting up a vicious circle. It is possible to rebalance your skin, however, and I have helped many people over the years with terrible skin problems.

Cleansing

Sleep, diet and exercise all contribute to a healthy-looking skin. Swapping your morning cup of coffee for some hot water with a squeeze of lemon will work wonders, as will fresh fruit juices. Facial exercises improve the

Oil-based cleanser for all skin types

Oil-based cleansers were used by many ancient cultures to cleanse and nourish the skin. This is a simple way of cleansing and has been known to me for many years. Depending on your skin type (see pages 80–83), invest in almond, wheatgerm, avocado, sunflower, borage or primrose oil. Aloe vera also works well.

Massage a small amount of your chosen oil into your face and neck using sweeping movements. Rub off with a dry flannel and follow with a hot compress (see below). This is an ideal way of cleaning the face. Do morning and night. All cleansers will keep for about one month. ❧

Cleansing oil for normal skin

80ml grapeseed oil
20ml (2 dessert spoons) almond oil
2 capsules wheatgerm oil
10 drops essential oil of lavender
100ml bottle

Add the ingredients to the bottle. Shake well. Pour a little of the cleanser into the palm of your hand and massage it around your chin, neck and décolleté in upward strokes. Use circular movements for the cheeks and around the eyes and lastly from the edge of the eyebrows to the scalp. Rub the cleanser off with a dry flannel using circular movements. Next add two drops of lavender to a washbasin of hot water. Submerge the flannel and squeeze out the excess before covering the face and

breathing deeply. Do this two or three times. After a hard day's work this is divine and so relaxing. All the tension will leave your body. ❧

Cleansing lotion for normal skin

½ bar of unperfumed, pH-balanced soap
60ml boiled water
30ml (2 tablespoons) soya oil
2 capsules wheatgerm oil
5 drops essential oil of either lavender or palmarosa
100ml bottle

Use a potato peeler to peel small strips of the soap. Transfer to the bottle with the rest of the ingredients. The cleansing lotion will be opaque and slightly soapy. Apply a little to the face with a damp cloth and rinse well with tepid water. Follow with the rose flower toner (see page 86). ❧

Cleansing oil for mature skin

This is a wonderful cleanser for mature skins. Alternate between rose, bois de rose, neroli, petit grain and orange essential oils; you need six drops in total.

45ml (3 tablespoons) almond oil
20ml (2 dessert spoons) jojoba oil
10ml (1 dessert spoon) castor oil
30ml (2 tablespoons) rose or marigold herbal tea or aloe vera juice
2 capsules borage oil
3 capsules evening primrose oil
3 capsules wheatgerm oil
3 drops essential oil of rose
3 drops essential oil of neroli
150ml bottle

Pour into the bottle and shake well. Place a little on a damp flannel, massaging it gently in. Remove with warm water then a cold rinse. ❧

Cleansing oil for dry skin

An oil-based cleanser is an absolute must for people suffering from dry skin! Good essential oils to use are myrrh, galbanum, bois de rose, rose, carrot, frankincense and patchouli. The recipe below requires six drops in total so feel free to alternate between these oils – try three drops of two different oils or six drops of one.

80ml avocado oil
10ml (1 dessert spoon) castor oil
5ml (1 teaspoon) jojoba oil
3 capsules borage oil
2 capsules wheatgerm oil
1 capsule evening primrose oil
3 drops essential oil of bois de rose
3 drops essential oil of frankincense
100ml bottle

Pour into the bottle and shake well. Follow instructions for cleansing before massaging the oil all over the face and on the nape of the neck. Dip a flannel in a washbasin of hot water and two drops of one of the oils described. Gently remove the excess oil with the flannel. Rinse with cold water followed by the chamomile and yarrow toner (see page 86). ❧

Cleansing oil for oily skin

Many people assume that you can't use oils on oily skins but in actual fact both the carrier oils and the essential oils help to rebalance the sebum secretions. It is important though to make sure you clean your hands thoroughly before cleansing as infections can easily spread. Oily skins need antiseptic oils such as basil, geranium, juniper, lemongrass and rosemary. You can alternate between them, mixing and matching to your tastes.

50ml grapeseed oil
50ml soya oil
1 capsule wheatgerm oil
15 drops essential oil of basil
15 drops essential oil of geranium
100ml bottle

Pour into the bottle and shake well. Follow instructions for cleansing before massaging the oil all over the face and on the nape of the neck. Dip a flannel in a washbasin of hot water and two drops of tea tree essential oil. Use this to gently remove the excess oil. Rinse with cold water followed by the chamomile toner (see page 86). ❧

Cleanser for oily skin

70ml grapeseed oil
30ml (2 tablespoons) sunflower oil
1 capsule wheatgerm oil
15 drops essential oil of either tea tree or rosemary
100ml bottle

Mix all the ingredients in the bottle and shake well. Follow instructions as for previous cleanser, substituting lavender in the final rinse for either tea tree or rosemary. ❧

Exfoliating

Many exfoliators and scrubs on the market today are too harsh and if used too often they can disrupt the skin's natural balance – the sebaceous glands will produce more sebum, making the skin oilier. You should only exfoliate once a week. Essential oils act as exfoliators but are a lot gentler, and if you mix them with oats and poppy or kiwi seeds you have a great natural scrub! Good essential oils to use are juniper, lemon, marjoram and peppermint – alternate them every time you make a new batch.

Gentle exfoliating mask for mature skin

Papaya contains natural enzymes that will gently digest dead skin cells and remove impurities.

1 fresh, ripe papaya, seeds removed
10ml (1 dessert spoon) almond oil
1 capsule wheatgerm oil
1 capsule borage oil
A few drops of freshly squeezed lemon juice

Use a spoon to scrape out the flesh of the papaya. Put in a blender with the rest of the ingredients. Blend to a pulp before applying it to the face. Massage in and leave on for a few minutes. Remove the mask with hot water and finish with a splash of cold water or the marigold and yarrow toner (see page 86). ❧

Gentle exfoliating mask for oily skin

2 large tablespoons of oats
1 ripe kiwi fruit, mashed
1 capsule wheatgerm oil
1 drop essential oil of juniper
1 drop essential oil of peppermint
A few drops of freshly squeezed lemon juice

In a small bowl, mix all the ingredients together adding a little water to obtain a paste. Make sure your face is clean (remove make-up with a hot flannel) before you apply the mask. Massage it in gently using circular movements – on the forehead, around the cheeks, nose, chin and neck. Leave the mask on for a few minutes before removing with warm water and a flannel. Finish with the chamomile toner (see page 86). ❧

Toning

If you have normal skin a toner is not generally needed. Most toners on the market contain alcohol and can leave the skin vulnerable, upsetting its natural balance. If you stick to a good cleansing regime, you'll find this is enough to keep your face looking good. However, many women will be used to using a toner so if you really miss one try the following. Use twice a day after cleansing.

Peppermint toner for normal skin

1 peppermint tea bag or 4–5 fresh leaves
250ml boiling water
250ml bottle

Add the tea bag or the leaves to a saucepan of boiling water. Take off the heat and leave to infuse for ten minutes. When cool transfer to a bottle; this will keep in the fridge for two to three days. Apply to the face with cotton wool. ஃ

Rose flower toner for normal skin
100ml boiled water
5 drops essential oil of rose
100ml bottle

Add to the bottle and leave to rest for a few days in a dark place. Apply to the face with cotton wool. This will keep for up to two weeks in the fridge. ஃ

Rose toner for normal skin
80g red or pink fragrant rose petals
75ml white wine vinegar
500ml distilled or mineral water
Large bottle

Mix together the vinegar and petals. Leave for a week but make sure you shake it from time to time. Strain off the vinegar and replace with the water. **Note:** If you leave out the water, the vinegar provides effective relief for sore throats – just gargle with it twice a day! This will keep for up to a month in the fridge. ஃ

Sage vinegar tonic for normal to oily skin
2 tablespoons fresh sage leaves, chopped
500ml pure red wine vinegar
Large bottle

Add the sage to the vinegar and leave for two weeks in a dark place. Then add a tablespoon to a medium glass (150ml) of water and use after cleansing. This tonic will keep for up to six weeks in a cool place. ஃ

Marigold and yarrow toner for mature skin
1 marigold flower head
1 teaspoon or 1 sachet of yarrow
500ml boiling water

In a small bowl, pour the boiling water on top of the herbs. Leave to infuse for five minutes. Leave to cool and apply as a toner. This will keep in the fridge for two to three days. ஃ

Chamomile and yarrow toner/facial spray for dry skin
1 chamomile tea bag or 4 flower heads
1 teaspoon or 1 sachet of yarrow
500ml boiling water

In a small bowl, pour the boiling water on top of the herbs. Leave to infuse for five minutes. Leave to cool and apply as a toner; alternatively you can transfer to a spray bottle as a quick and easy way of hydrating your skin as often as needed. This will keep in the fridge for two to three days. ஃ

Chamomile toner for oily skin
1 chamomile tea bag or 4 flower heads
100ml water
3 drops essential oil of tea tree
100ml bottle

Add the tea bag or the flower heads to a saucepan of boiling water. Take off the heat and leave to infuse for five to ten minutes. When cool transfer to a bottle and add the tea tree essential oil. It will keep in the fridge for up to a week. Apply to the face with cotton wool, paying particular attention to the greasiest areas with the most open pores. ஃ

Aniseed skin toner for oily skin
Boil 2 teaspoons of aniseeds in 500ml water for 10 minutes. Let it cool for 20 minutes then pour into a bottle. Use as a skin toner twice a day. This will keep in the fridge for a week. ஃ

Moisturizing
A good massage twice a day with a moisturizing oil or cream will not only help the essential oils to be absorbed, delivering nutrients, but will also help the circulation and slow the development of wrinkles. Massage the oil in a circular movement around the sinus area and over the cheeks. Gently rub across the forehead before stroking the oil up the neck. You can also slightly pinch the oil into the nape of the neck. Most of the following oils will keep for up to two months.

Moisturizing face oil for normal skin
People who are lucky enough to have normal skin will benefit from using almond, sunflower or jojoba as carrier oils. Good essential oils to use are chamomile, lavender, palmarosa, grapefruit and bois de rose. With

these as a base you can make bespoke moisturizers every time, tailoring the oils to your tastes (every two months change either the essential oils or carrier oil) and your skin will reap the benefits. In the recipe below, I've used almond oil but you could also try jojoba or sunflower. The two essential oils can also be mixed and matched with any of the above.

50ml almond oil
2 capsules borage oil
2 capsules wheatgerm oil
4 drops essential oil of chamomile
4 drops essential oil of bois de rose
100ml bottle

Mix the ingredients together in the bottle and shake well. Apply this oil to your face after cleansing. ᴄᴀ

Moisturizing face cream for normal skin

50ml pot fragrance-free (organic if possible) moisturizing cream
3 drops of your chosen essential oil

Use a spatula to mix the cream and oil together. Apply as directed above. ᴄᴀ

Moisturizing face mask for normal skin

Even normal skin can look dull and lifeless at times so use a face mask (after cleansing) once a week to help refine the pores and improve colour and texture. This treatment is especially good during the winter months – central heating can dry out the skin, causing it to become sensitive and susceptible to infection.

1 tablespoon white clay powder
3–4 tablespoons warm boiled water
1 capsule wheatgerm oil
1 capsule evening primrose oil
5ml (1 teaspoon) almond oil
3 drops essential oil of lavender, chamomile or palmarosa

Use a spatula to mix all the ingredients together to form a paste. Apply to the face and neck using circular movements to improve circulation. Leave the mask on for three to five minutes before removing with warm water. Finish by covering your face with a hot flannel infused with one of the oils from the mask ingredients. Moisturize face as normal. ᴄᴀ

Moisturizing face oil for mature skin

Massage the oil into your skin, as this will improve the muscle tone, increasing firmness and elasticity. It will make the muscles relax and the gentle exercise will slow sagging around the jaw line. We often forget that it is the muscles underneath the surface that give the face shape and contour. The essential oils and carrier oils described here will revitalize and provoke the return of the soft cushion that envelops the face, making it appear much younger and smoother.

Good essential oils for mature skins are rose, bois de rose, neroli, petit grain and orange. Ten drops are needed in total so you can alternate each time.

20ml (2 dessert spoons) avocado oil
15ml (1 tablespoon) almond oil
5ml (1 teaspoon) flax oil
5ml (1 teaspoon) jojoba oil
3 capsules wheatgerm oil
8 drops essential oil of rose
2 drops essential oil of orange
50ml bottle

Mix ingredients together and shake well. Apply to face twice a day, massaging in. ᴄᴀ

Moisturizing face cream for mature skin

If you would prefer a cream to an oil, this recipe is just as easy. You need to buy a simple, fragrance-free moisturizing cold cream as a base.

50ml pot fragrance-free moisturizing cold cream
5ml (1 teaspoon) jojoba oil
2 capsules wheatgerm oil
1 capsule evening primrose oil
3 drops essential oil of rose, bois de rose, neroli, petit grain or orange

Add all the ingredients to the cold cream and mix together with a spatula. Apply twice a day. ᴄᴀ

Geranium face oil for mature skin

10ml (1 dessert spoon) argan oil
20ml (2 dessert spoons) avocado oil
2 capsules borage oil
12 drops essential oil of geranium
2 drops essential oil of rose
1 drop essential oil of lemon
50ml bottle

Mix ingredients together and shake

well. Gently rub a drop of the oil into the face every evening. Do this for four to six weeks. ❧

Palmarosa face oil for mature skin

2 capsules wheatgerm oil
5ml (1 teaspoon) argan oil
5ml (1 teaspoon) avocado oil
5ml (1 teaspoon) rose masqueta oil
10ml (1 dessert spoon) almond oil
15 drops essential oil of palmarosa
3 drops essential oil of rose
2 drops essential oil of mint
50ml bottle

Mix well and apply to face at night – rub a little oil into the skin until absorbed, apply again. Do this every day for between three to six months. ❧

Moisturizing treatment for dry skin

This is a wonderful treatment to rebalance the skin secretions.

20g organic beeswax
60ml avocado oil
10ml (1 dessert spoon) jojoba oil
2 capsules wheatgerm oil
1 capsule evening primrose oil
1 capsule borage oil
10ml (1 dessert spoon) yarrow decoc-
    tion (see page 11)
6 drops (or 3 drops of 2) essential oil
    of rose, myrrh, galbanum, bois de
    rose, carrot, clary sage, peppermint,
    frankincense or patchouli
100ml jar

Use a bain-marie (see page 12) to warm up the beeswax. When melted, stir in the avocado and jojoba oils.

Leave to cool a little before adding the wheatgerm, evening primrose and borage oils. Pour into a mixing bowl, stirring until the mixture starts to thicken and change colour (it will become more opaque). Slowly mix in the yarrow decoction, adding it a little at a time. Add your chosen essential oil and transfer to a jar. Apply this treatment at night when your skin is at its most relaxed. Store in the fridge. ❧

Moisturizing face oil for dry skin

45ml (3 tablespoons) almond oil
5ml (1 teaspoon) argan oil
2 capsules wheatgerm oil
8 drops essential oil of lavender
2 drops essential oil of bois de rose
1 drop essential oil of chamomile
50ml bottle

Mix ingredients together. Apply this oil after cleansing in the evening. When the first application has absorbed into the skin, apply another. ❧

Moisturizing gel mask for dry skin

1 tablespoon slippery elm powder
A little boiled water
A small cup of cold chamomile tea
10ml (1 dessert spoon) castor oil
1 capsule borage oil
1 capsule evening primrose oil
2 drops essential oil of rose, myrrh,
    galbanum, bois de rose, carrot,
    frankincense, clary sage,
    peppermint or patchouli

In a small saucepan, mix the slippery elm powder with a little water to

obtain a paste. Pour in the chamomile tea and slowly bring to the boil until the mixture thickens. Leave the mask to cool, before adding the castor, borage and evening primrose oils, and the essential oil of your choice. Apply the mask to your face after cleansing. Leave for a few minutes. Wipe off with a hot compress. Use once or twice a month. ❧

Moisturizing oat and linseed mask for dry skin

2 tablespoons linseeds, crushed
2 tablespoons oats
A glass of hot water
3 drops essential oil of rose, myrrh,
    galbanum, bois de rose, carrot,
    frankincense, clary sage,
    peppermint or patchouli
2 A4 size pieces of gauze
2 cotton wool pads

First grind the linseeds in a blender. Add to a saucepan with the oats and slowly add the water to obtain a paste. Bring to the boil stirring well. Leave to cool before adding your chosen essential oil. Place the two pieces of gauze on a washable surface (make sure they're portrait like a piece of A4 paper) and fold the left edges over to the right edges, unfold again. Use a spatula to spread the paste along (and either side of) the central line. Now fold into quarters. Lie down on your bed and place the cotton wool pads over each eye before covering your forehead with one of the masks. Place the other one over the lower part of your face leaving your nose exposed. (This part is tricky and you may need someone else to help you.) Relax for ten minutes. Finish with the chamomile and yarrow toner (see page 86). Then moisturize as normal. Use once a month. ᐦ

Orange pick-me-up face mask for dry skin

50ml pure orange juice
2 tablespoons white clay powder
1 capsule wheatgerm oil
5ml (1 teaspoon) argan oil
8 drops essential oil of orange
100ml jar

Mix well with a spatula and transfer to a glass jar. Apply to the face and neck once or twice a week. Leave on for five to seven minutes until set, removing with warm water. This will keep for about a month in the fridge. ᐦ

Rejuvenating face mask

2 tablespoons white clay powder
½ cup cold chamomile tea
5ml (1 teaspoon) argan oil
1 capsule wheatgerm oil
6 drops essential oil of palmarosa

Mix well with a spatula. Use the mask on your face twice a week – leave on until set, removing with warm water and finishing with a cold flannel. ᐦ

Rejuvenating face oil with sage for dry skin

10ml (1 dessert spoon) almond oil
10ml (1 dessert spoon) grapeseed oil
1 capsule wheatgerm oil
1 capsule borage oil
5 drops essential oil of clary sage
1 drop essential oil of mint

2 drops essential oil of chamomile
50ml bottle

Mix and massage into face twice a day after cleansing. This will help relax tense facial muscles. The combination of clary sage and mint will refresh and decongest, relaxing the face. ᐦ

Gel moisturizer for oily skin

Gels are good for most skins but excellent for oily skins. They are cheap to make and extremely effective. I like to use pectin, which comes from apple peel. This is available is most health food shops but if you're feeling motivated you can always make your own: peel four or five apples and put the skins into a small saucepan with two heads of chamomile. Cover with water and bring to the boil very slowly. Cook for up to forty-five minutes until the liquid has reduced by one-third. Strain and return to the saucepan to simmer until you obtain a concentrate. When this cools it will turn to gel and you can use it in this recipe.

1 tablespoon pectin powder (see page 8)
50ml water
5ml (1 teaspoon) grapeseed oil
5 drops essential oil of tea tree, basil, geranium, juniper, lemongrass or rosemary
50g pot

Add enough water to the pectin powder to get a paste. Then mix the grapeseed oil with the pectin. Add the

essential oil of your choice and mix again. Apply as needed once or twice a day. This gel is very soothing and slightly astringent – wonderful for acne. It will keep for up to a month in the fridge. ᐦ

Moisturizing face oil for oily skin

This special face oil contains essential oils that have the capacity to help rebalance the sebum secretions. Alternate between grapeseed and soya oils and the essential oils described in the moisturizing gel for oily skin, above.

45ml (3 tablespoons) grapeseed oil
10ml (1 dessert spoon) jojoba oil
1 capsule evening primrose oil
1 capsule wheatgerm oil
6 drops essential oil of juniper
6 drops essential oil of geranium
100ml bottle

Pour into the bottle and shake well. Massage the oil gently into the face and neck, taking the surplus off with a damp flannel. ᐦ

Moisturizing face oil for oily skin

50ml soya oil
1 capsule wheatgerm oil
10 drops essential oil of lavender
3 drops essential oil of cypress
50ml bottle

Mix ingredients together. Apply this oil after cleansing in the evening. When the first application has absorbed, apply a second one. ᐦ

BEFORE AND AFTER COSMETIC SURGERY

I firmly believe that if people look after their skin and themselves, through a good diet and plenty of exercise, they shouldn't need to resort to cosmetic surgery.

For others, however, cosmetic surgery can change their lives by altering a feature or condition that has caused them to suffer low self-esteem for years. Whatever the reason for opting for surgery, essential oils can do a great deal to prepare skin and to help with the healing process afterwards. Any decision about whether or not to undergo cosmetic surgery should be considered seriously as there are many risks involved. Remember that it is important to have all the procedures explained to you beforehand as you need to know what to expect and whether there could be any complications. Make sure you are really comfortable with everything before you go ahead.

The after-effects of cosmetic surgery can vary from person to person and health, skin quality, age and gender will all play a part. The most common problem will be swelling and bruising, although reactions to drugs and anaesthetics are not unusual. Afterwards you will be asked to look out for signs of infection, blood clots (haematoma) or accumulating fluid (seroma). There may also be temporary nerve problems, especially on the face, and numbness can be felt for a few months. Some people will also experience bad scarring.

The decision to have cosmetic surgery can be hard both emotionally and psychologically. But once you've made the decision to go ahead, it is extremely important to look after your skin very carefully for at least six weeks before surgery. Essential oils are fantastic for helping to keep the elasticity and texture of the skin, removing toxins and rehydrating. Follow the cleansing and moisturizing recipes given in the book for dry skin and you will reap the benefits. The following oil is particularly good for nourishing the skin beforehand.

Before surgery
Protecting face oil
This oil is particularly good for more mature skin.

30ml (2 tablespoons) rose masqueta oil
10ml (1 dessert spoon) avocado oil
10ml (1 dessert spoon) jojoba oil
2 capsules wheatgerm oil
5 drops essential oil of rose
2 drops essential oil of galbanum
1 drop essential oil of peppermint
50ml bottle

Mix ingredients together in the bottle and use a little to massage into the face and front of the neck, ears and back of the neck. Concentrate particularly around the hairline and behind the ears where the skin will be pulled. Use every evening when your skin is at its most relaxed. This oil will keep for two to three months. ❧

Face oil to protect against scarring
50ml avocado oil
10ml (1 dessert spoon) argan oil
1 capsule wheatgerm oil
2 capsules borage oil
12 drops essential oil of rose
8 drops essential oil of bois de rose
100ml bottle

Mix ingredients together in the bottle and massage face, neck, forehead and behind the ears twice a day for six weeks before the operation. This oil will keep for two to three months. ❧

De-stress bath

There will always be apprehension before any kind of surgery so it is important to try and relax. Good oils to use are neroli, rose, petit grain, lavender and jasmine. Choose one and add three to five drops to the running water. Relax for up to fifteen minutes. ॐ

De-stress body oil

This will help relax you and is excellent either after the bath above or on its own.

50ml soya oil
50ml jojoba oil
2 capsules wheatgerm oil
5 drops essential oil of rose or jasmine
5 drops essential oil of petit grain
   or neroli
100ml bottle

Mix ingredients together in the bottle and massage into the torso and the neck. ॐ

Rose and peppermint pre-surgery facial spray

Make an infusion from a handful of rose petals (you can buy these dried from health food shops) and half a handful of fresh peppermint leaves in 600ml (1 pint) of boiling water. Leave to cool, strain and pour into a spray bottle. Spray your face with this a few times a day. Using this will prepare the skin for surgery – it will help maintain elasticity, increase suppleness and hydration – all making the surgeon's work easier! This will keep fresh for two to three days. ॐ

After surgery

After surgery the skin will be extra-sensitive, tight, swollen and bruised; some scars will also be forming. You have to be patient at this time as there is a risk of infection but if the surgeon has properly advised you and monitored your progress, you will hopefully have few problems.

When your skin is recovering, you can return to the same products that you used before surgery, especially the face oil (see the section in the book on dry skin too, page 82). Compresses are advised, as are linseed and oatmeal poultices (but not too hot). (See page 12.) Stay away from facial massage for a while until your skin has completely recovered and it will take time for the numbness to disappear. Also keep out of the sun and invest in a humidifier which will help your skin recover and scars to heal. Try walking outside when it rains.

Healing black pepper oil

This oil is good for revitalizing the skin, strengthening muscle tone and relieving numbness.

50ml rose masqueta oil
10ml (1 dessert spoon) jojoba oil
1 capsule wheatgerm oil
1 capsule evening primrose oil
1 capsule borage oil
6 drops essential oil of black pepper
3 drops essential oil of galbanum
3 drops essential oil of rose
2 drops essential oil of frankincense
100ml bottle

Mix ingredients together in the bottle and shake well. Massage gently into the skin twice a day after cleansing. This oil will keep for two to three months. ॐ

Tea tree cream for scars

25g organic beeswax
70ml almond oil
5ml (1 teaspoon) jojoba oil
1 capsule wheatgerm oil
15 drops essential oil of tea tree
5 drops essential oil of palmarosa
2 drops essential oil of chamomile
Jar

Warm up the beeswax in a bain-marie (see page 12). When melted, add the almond, wheatgerm and jojoba oils. Beat them together. Take off the heat and leave to cool for a while before adding the essential oils. Put into a glass jar, applying twice a day after cleansing. This cream will keep for up to three months. ॐ

Skin problems

The skin is a window to the general health of the body and any changes taking place within will show up on its surface. Many skin problems are a result of bad diet, stress, reactions to drugs or even skin-care products. For instance, skin bleaching products and chemical peels can cause terrible problems – burns, cracks and eczema are common, which is a high price to pay for looking good. Many women also experience a bout of spots just before a period.

Strong drugs and ointments are often prescribed for conditions such as eczema and acne but in fact they prevent the skin's natural process of elimination and can exacerbate problems in the long term as toxins cannot be processed through the skin. A natural approach to treatment is preferable so try and avoid stimulants such as coffee, tea and chocolate, which can activate sebum secretions and thus cause spots, replacing them with herbal teas and fresh juices, which are naturally cleansing. Dairy products can sometimes aggravate skin problems too. Just as important is to try to remain calm and free from stress as this too can cause a build-up of sebum secretions. Essential oils will help problem skins in a gentle way and can give wonderful results if you use them regularly.

Acne amd acne rosacea

Acne is a disorder of the sebaceous glands, often caused by a hormone imbalance, causing spots, blackheads and small abscesses. The blocked pores get infected, sometimes with the bacterium staphylococcus, and the surface of the skin becomes inflamed and painful. Acne can develop on the parts of the skin where the glands are in great numbers, such as the nose, chin and forehead. Many people use strong drugs and powerful cleansing treatments to try and help the situation but these tend to remove every trace of the skin's natural, protecting oils. The result is more sebum secretions, creating more spots! I have treated acne for years and know how difficult it can be for teenagers and adults alike. Sometimes it corrects itself after the mid-twenties but I have often seen women in their thirties with this condition.

Acne rosacea has similar symptoms to and is often mistaken for regular acne. It is characterized by a permanent redness and skin inflammation, and those afflicted tend to blush easily. It is associated with excessive oiliness and mostly appears on the nose and cheeks. It should be treated with the same preparations as those for acne and special attention should be paid to cleansing.

Essential oils will restore the natural balance of the sebaceous glands. Their antibiotic properties and natural plant hormones will correct hormone imbalances and help reduce the unpleasant symptoms, banishing spots, healing scars and easing inflammation.

Acne treatment
50ml soya oil
1 capsule evening primrose oil
1 capsule wheatgerm oil
15 drops essential oil of lavender
3 drops essential oil of bois de rose
50ml bottle

Mix ingredients together in the bottle and gently massage this lovely oil into the face after cleansing. When the first application is absorbed, apply a second one. Use once a day, in the evening. This oil will keep for up to two months. ❧

Peppermint face oil for acne/open pores
20ml (2 dessert spoons) almond oil
2 capsules wheatgerm oil
5ml (1 teaspoon) grapeseed oil
15 drops essential oil of peppermint
6 drops essential oil of cypress
6 drops essential oil of chamomile
50ml bottle

Mix ingedients together in the bottle. Apply to the face morning and night after cleansing – massage a little into the face and, when absorbed, apply again.

Continue treatment for a few months or until the skin is clear and refined. It will keep for up to two months. ∿

Astringent toner for large pores

Juice of ¹/₂ cucumber, peeled
100ml rosewater
3 drops essential oil of lemon
1 drop essential oil of carrot
¹/₂ litre bottle

Use a liquidizer to obtain a cucumber pulp and then strain through a sieve (if you have a juicer, all the better!). Mix the ingredients together. Apply to affected areas twice a day after cleansing. This will keep for up to ten days in the fridge. ∿

Clay mask for enlarged pores

This is a great treatment for use once or twice a week, depending on the severity of your condition. It will tone the skin, reducing the size of the open pores.

1 tablespoon green clay powder
A little boiled water
A few drops freshly squeezed lemon juice
2 drops essential oil of either juniper or tea tree

Mix the clay with a little boiled water to obtain a paste. Add the lemon juice and your chosen essential oil. Apply the mask to the affected areas and leave on for five minutes. Remove with warm water, finishing with a cold rinse. Follow with an application of one of the toners recommended for oily skin (see page 86). ∿

Blackheads and whiteheads

Black/whiteheads are small black or yellow plugs on the skin that are caused by a build-up of oil in the pore. Oils that help include lavender, lemon, palmarosa, patchouli and lemongrass. Try experimenting with each one, alternating each time.

Steam treatment for black/whiteheads

Steaming is an excellent way to loosen these small plugs. It opens the pores and disinfects the area to make it ready for squeezing.

Gently steam your face over a bowl of just boiled water containing a drop of your chosen oil from the list above. Cover your head with a towel for a few minutes. Next, dissolve one tablespoon Epsom salts in a bowl of hot water. Add three drops of your oil. Soak a small flannel in the solution, wring it slightly then press it to your face rubbing the area around the blackhead gently. Repeat a few times then use a tissue to carefully squeeze out the blackhead – do not force the stubborn ones; wait until next time. Finish with an aloe vera solution made by mixing one tablespoon of organic aloe vera juice with one drop of essential oil of lemongrass. Apply to the skin where the blackhead was. ∿

Face oil for blackheads

Put a few drops of essential oil of geranium in a bowl of boiling water (200ml will suffice). Cover your head with a towel and place your face above

the bowl so you can feel the vapours on your skin. This will open the pores.

Follow with a gentle massage with the following oil:

30ml (2 tablespoons) soya oil
1 capsule wheatgerm oil
15 drops essential oil of geranium
2 drops essential oil of sandalwood
50ml bottle

Mix ingredients together in the bottle and shake well. Use twice a week. This oil will keep for up to two months. This is particularly good for acne sufferers too. ∿

Skin lightening

I don't advise bleaching the skin with strong chemicals as they can cause irreparable damage. Lemon juice or buttermilk is much gentler and better for the skin if you want to achieve a lighter skin colour.

Lightening gel

¹/₂ dessertspoon pectin powder (see page 8)
A little boiled water
5ml (1 teaspoon) castor oil
Freshly squeezed juice of ¹/₂ lemon
2 drops essential oil of lemon
Jar

In a mug, dissolve the pectin powder in a little boiled water. Add the castor oil, lemon juice and essential oil of lemon. Mix and place in the fridge, covered, for a few hours. Massage into the face and neck, morning and night, after cleansing. This gel can be kept for up to ten days in the fridge. ∿

Buttermilk lightening recipe

Buttermilk is an excellent natural, gentle bleach and this recipe is good for the hands too.

150ml buttermilk
10ml (1 dessert spoon) cider vinegar
100ml rosewater or a rose petal
    infusion made with half-a-handful
    of petals (see page 11)
1/2 effervescent vitamin C tablet
    (widely available from chemists)
15ml (1 tablespoon) freshly squeezed
    lemon juice
1 drop essential oil of lemon
1/2 litre bottle

Mix all the ingredients together and pour into a bottle. Apply to the face with a small sponge; it will absorb. Apply a second and third time before rinsing face with warm water. Finish with a toner such as rosewater or lavender water. Use two to three times a week. The lotion will keep for two to three days in the fridge. ✍

Ageing spots

These brownish marks can occur on the hands, arms and face and are associated with ageing and over-exposure to the sun.

Fading treatment for ageing spots

10ml (1 dessert spoon) castor oil
10ml (1 dessert spoon) cranberry juice
1 drop essential oil of either
    sandalwood or galbanum
Jar

Mix together in a small jar. Apply to affected areas once a day using a

cotton bud. This will keep for two to three weeks in the fridge. ✍

Broken capillaries/ spider veins

These are often associated with fair, delicate skins that burn easily in the sun. They are especially noticeable on the cheeks and décolleté. Avoid hot baths and showers, hot facials, the sun and alcohol as all these things cause the capillaries to dilate. Vitamin C in your diet is important, as is rutin (found in the pith that surrounds citrus fruits). Both are extremely good for strengthening the walls of veins.

Parsley is also a particularly effective essential oil to use as it slows down the spread of broken capillaries and reduces their appearance. I have also found essential oils of chamomile, violet leaves and orange to be good.

Face oil for broken capillaries

30ml (2 tablespoons) rose masqueta
    oil
10ml (1 dessert spoon) argan oil
2 capsules borage oil
2 capsules wheatgerm oil
6 drops essential oil of parsley
2 drops essential oil of chamomile,
    violet leaves or orange
50ml bottle

Mix together in the bottle and gently apply to the face after cleansing, preferably in the morning. After ten minutes, remove any surplus oil with a tissue. This oil will keep for two to three months. ✍

Parsley tonic

Juice enough fresh parley to fill one-quarter of a small (100ml) glass. Fill the rest of the glass with boiled water and add one drop of essential oil of parsley. Transfer to a bottle and apply after the face oil each morning. This can be kept in the fridge for a week to ten days. ✍

Facial puffiness

There are many possible causes for a puffy face, the most serious being some forms of kidney disease, but the most common are the contraceptive pill, pregnancy, PMS, food allergies and fluid retention. Always check with your doctor if symptoms persist.

Toner to reduce puffiness

Chamomile and comfrey are both skin-healing herbs. Use a teapot to make this quick toner.

3 fresh heads chamomile or 1 tea bag
    or 1 dessertspoon comfrey
100ml boiling water
Teapot

Cover your chosen herb in boiling water and leave to infuse for ten minutes. When cool, apply to your face with cotton wool. No need to rinse. Alternatively, you can dampen a piece of gauze in the solution and use it as a face compress. Leave on for a few minutes. Use twice a day when the condition is bad, then two to three times a week until puffiness is reduced. Make up a fresh solution each time. ✍

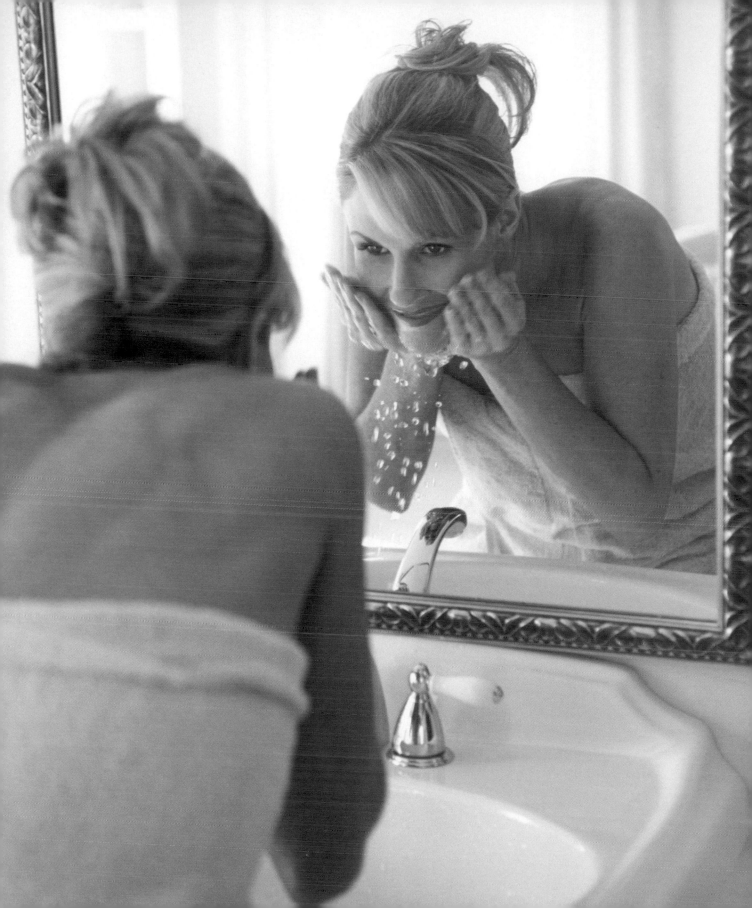

EASING THE MENSTRUAL CYCLE

The menstrual cycle begins at puberty and continues through the heart of a woman's life, stopping at the menopause, and only interrupted during pregnancy and breastfeeding.

The whole cycle usually takes about twenty-eight days, although it is not abnormal for it to last longer (or shorter); it varies from woman to woman.

Menstruation affects women in different ways – some are beset with many problems while others hardly notice their periods. But the majority will experience some upheaval – a consequence of continual fluctuations in hormone levels. For a few days or weeks each month, these problems can impact heavily on a woman's life and many will want to find a solution.

During a woman's period her sense of smell will alter. The nerve cells in the nasal passages are directly linked to the region of the brain that influences the pituitary gland (the limbic region). This has a direct link to the reproductive system and an impact on the quantities of oestrogen and progesterone produced. Research carried out by Dr Wilhelm Fliess in Germany suggests that a woman's menstrual cycle can be affected by different smells and pheromones (chemicals that transmit messages). It has also been noted that the pheromones a woman produces (found on skin, hair and in bodily secretions) change throughout her cycle. Her sense of smell becomes more sensitive before and during a period, too, only getting back to normal after her period. This may indicate that if essential oils (containing natural plant hormones) are applied, inhaled or vaporized at different times throughout the menstrual cycle, they can have a hugely positive influence.

Essential oils can ease menstrual symptoms; since they are natural diuretics and induce relaxation. Just a simple inhalation, bath or massage with an oil can make all the difference.

Pre-menstrual syndrome (PMS)

When the female hormones (oestrogen and progesterone) are in perfect balance we feel healthy and well, both mentally and physically. But when, for example, an inadequate amount of progesterone is released prior to menstruation, the release of the other hormones is disrupted. It is this imbalance that is thought to be the cause of PMS. (In recent years, many women have experienced an increase in their oestrogen levels, known as oestrogen dominance. This makes them prone to menstrual and menopausal problems, and recent research has linked it to cancer. Some think that the contraceptive pill is a factor; others suggest that oestrogen has somehow entered the food chain. The true cause has yet to be established.) A lack of certain vitamins, especially the B vitamins, is also thought to be a cause of PMS and many women are prescribed them to alleviate the symptoms.

The symptoms of PMS include personality changes (assertive and outgoing one minute, submissive and introspective the next), stomach cramps, breast pain, backache, fatigue, insomnia, bloating and fluid retention, constipation, skin problems and headaches. Some women will experience a change in their appetite; others may weep for no apparent reason.

Many women resort to one of the numerous diuretics on the market in the hope that they will banish excess fluid and bloating. But these will cause many important minerals, such as potassium, to be lost and this will result in feelings of even greater fatigue.

Keeping symptoms under control

There are a number of different steps you can take that will be beneficial and may remove some of the symptoms. Firstly, avoid stimulants such as coffee, tea and alcohol, as these will interfere with the body's absorption of vitamins. Instead replace them with calming herbal teas such as linden (tilleul, lime blossom), chamomile, orange leaves, verbena (vervein), fennel, feverfew and aniseed.

Try to eat regularly, especially small snacks that are rich in vitamin B complex and vitamin B6. These essential vitamins are found in whole grains, nuts, meat (especially liver), oily fish, sprouting seeds, soya beans and avocados. Magnesium is also good for PMS so include grapes and oats in your diet. Eating sensibly and regularly is essential, as it will keep your blood sugar at a constant level. Taking evening primrose oil can also help.

During a period the sebaceous glands are more active and the skin may become more oily. Spots and blemishes can appear suddenly so change your skin care regime to reflect this. Try the remedies for oily skin instead of your usual type.

All in all, you can alleviate many of the symptoms by changing your skin routine, taking relaxing, aromatic baths and using massage oils.

Essential oils

There are many essential oils that will help alleviate the symptoms of PMS and other menstrual problems. Alternate between them, making a note of how you respond and changing them accordingly.

Basil – helps the nervous system, headaches.

Bergamot – helps loss of appetite.

Bois de rose – general stimulant.

Calendula – good for the skin, relaxes.

Caraway – helps pain.

Celery – slightly diuretic.

Chamomile – alleviates fluid retention, rebalances hormones.

Clary sage – eases stress.

Cypress – decongesting, eases heavy sweating, circulatory problems.

Geranium – a nerve tonic, calms urinary infections.

Ginger – combats fatigue.

Lavender – aids relaxation.

Lemongrass – helps headaches and migraine, analgesic.

Mandarin – helps nervous tension.

Marjoram – a tonic for the nervous system.

Melissa – aids relaxation, helps the nervous system.

Neroli – helps nervous tension.

Nutmeg – helps with pre-menstrual pain, blood circulation.

Oregano – has anti-fatigue, anti-stress properties.

Palmarosa – rebalances skin secretions.

Parsley – a wonderful oil during period time. Helps eliminate pain and fluid retention.

Peppermint – analgesic, helps headaches, decongestive.

Petit grain – helps nervous tension.

Ravensare/Ravensara – eases backache, fatigue.

Rose – helps regulate and rebalance the cycle.

Sandalwood – eases bloating before a period.

Thyme – has anti-fatigue, anti-stress properties.

Verbena (vervein) – good for palpitations, depression.

Bath essence for aches and pains

Keep your bath to body temperature, no hotter. Alternate between rose and palmarosa, thyme and clary sage, fennel and celery oils.

45ml (3 tablespoons) grapeseed oil
1 capsule wheatgerm oil
1 capsule evening primrose oil
6 drops essential oil of chamomile
12 drops essential oil of cypress
10 drops essential oil of parsley
12 drops essential oil of petit grain
5 drops essential oil of either rose or palmarosa
12 drops essential oil of either thyme or clary sage
10 drops essential oil of either fennel or celery
50ml bottle

Mix ingredients together. Use 1 tablespoon of the essence per bath (mix it with a little fragrance-free bubble bath), pouring under running water. Relax for 10 minutes. This will keep for up to 6 weeks in a cool place. ❧

Massage oil for aches and pains

A massage with this oil will be wonderful after your bath. You can alternate between the oils suggested.

20ml (2 dessert spoons) almond oil
1 capsule wheatgerm oil
1 capsule evening primrose oil
6 drops essential oil of either nutmeg or ravensare
6 drops essential oil of either verbena or lemongrass
4 drops essential oil of parsley

2 drops essential oil of peppermint
50ml bottle

Mix ingredients together in the bottle and shake well. Rub a little over your stomach area and solar plexus in a clockwise direction. Massage the lower part of your back. Use daily for about a week. This oil will keep for two to three months. ❧

Amenorrhoea

Amenorrhoea indicates an absence of menstruation during puberty although it is not uncommon for a young girl to experience irregular periods to start with. This condition is more of a health concern if experienced during later life. Some women will cease menstruating if they suffer from anorexia nervosa as the body is deprived of many important nutrients (a lack of vitamins A, E, F and B complex, and zinc all contribute to amenorrhoea). I have also treated women whose periods have stopped due to an emotional shock, only to return months later when their condition has improved. Long distance air travel can also be a cause and many airhostesses find their periods are absent as their body clocks are in constant turmoil. Tisanes will help this condition and both sage and chamomile are helpful.

Bath treatment

If the amenorrhoea is the result of an emotional problem it will eventually return to normal. However, essential oils could be of benefit and encourage the cycle to start again. Chamomile,

neroli, clary sage, parsley and cypress are all good. Choose two and add 5 drops of each to a bath. ❧

Massage oil

Again choose two of the above oils. Add a drop of each to 10ml (1 dessert spoon) of almond oil. Use this to massage the solar plexus and tummy in circular movements. Use daily for a week. ❧

Dysmenorrhoea

These are the painful, cramping periods suffered by many women. The cramps can be quite violent and uncomfortable, and can worsen under severe anxiety and stress. The condition is sometimes accompanied by urine infections. Before a period starts, a woman will experience bloating and fluid retention, back pain and cramps in the pelvic area – not fun! Drink tisanes (see page 11) of peppermint, liquorice root, ginger, chamomile and verbena (vervein).

Massage oil

Good oils to use for this are nutmeg, lavender, peppermint, chamomile, ravensare and verbena. Always make it with nutmeg but alternate the others. Here I've used chamomile and lavender.

30ml (2 tablespoons) soya oil
20ml (2 dessert spoons) almond oil
2 capsules evening primrose oil
1 capsule wheatgerm oil
10 drops essential oil of nutmeg
8 drops essential oil of chamomile
8 drops essential oil of lavender
100ml bottle

Mix together in the bottle and shake well. Rub this oil on the abdomen, solar plexus, lower back, nape of the neck and shoulders, top of the hands and along the arms towards the heart. If you have bad stomach cramps, put a couple of drops of the oil on a tissue and place on the stomach, a hot water bottle on top. Lie down and relax for twenty minutes with the feet elevated. Use daily for a week. The oil will keep for up to six weeks. ❧

Menorrhagia

These are abnormally heavy and prolonged periods with clots. They can also be irregular. If you suffer from menorrhagia it is important to consult your doctor to make sure there isn't a more serious underlying condition. Essential oils can be extremely beneficial, have aromatic baths and regular massages.

Bath and massage oil

30ml (2 tablespoons) soya oil
1 capsule wheatgerm oil
1 capsule evening primrose oil
10 drops essential oil of clary sage
10 drops essential oil of chamomile
10 drops essential oil of palmarosa or geranium
50ml bottle

Mix together in the bottle and use one capful per bath. Alternatively, pour a little of the oil into the palm of your hand and massage your abdomen in a clockwise direction until absorbed. This oil will keep for two to three months. ❧

HAVING A POSITIVE MENOPAUSE

Most women in the Western world view the menopause with great apprehension in the belief that the loss of their fertility will go hand in hand with the loss of sexuality, beauty and youthfulness.

But menopause is simply the end of the menstrual cycle, just as puberty was its start.

It usually occurs between the ages of 42–50 but some women can experience it in their 30s. Gradually the ovaries will cease to respond to the stimulation of the female hormones. Periods and pain will stop and with them the suffering, women can enjoy a normal sex life without the need for contraception. Some people sail through the menopause with little discomfort, for others it is not so easy.

Symptoms of the menopause include irritability, nervousness, stiffness, aches and pains, insomnia, palpitations, rashes and itchy skin. High blood pressure, depression and headaches can also appear, as can hot flushes. These can cause embarrassment and discomfort as suddenly you feel so sweaty and your face becomes red. The menopause is a good time to get a full health check, especially if you suffer from high blood pressure or palpitations. Get your cholesterol levels checked too.

HRT is regularly prescribed to alleviate some of the worse symptoms. Its job is to replace the lost hormones but I feel that many women would be better off without it. Many symptoms are manageable and more so if you eat fresh fruit and vegetables. Food rich in plant hormones are especially good – soya products, yams, papayas and cucumbers. Organic seeds and grains, and seaweeds can also be beneficial, as can royal jelly, pollen, evening primrose oil, wheatgerm oil and Manuka honey. Avoid spicy foods and stimulants if you suffer from hot flushes or palpitations.

Herbal teas are a must. Make tisanes of orange leaves, sage, verbena, angelica, rosemary, thyme, liquorice root, jasmine or melissa. Nettle and chamomile are particularly good. Exercise regularly too; this boosts the circulation and eases depression.

Essential oils can influence a sluggish system and assist during hard times. They help soothe emotions too. Good ones to try include:

Angelica – good for all the symptoms.
Aniseed – counteracts fluid retention, helps palpitations and calms nervousness.
Cardamom – diuretic, helps fluid retention.
Chamomile – calms and soothes.
Clary sage – helps calm anxiety, reduces swelling and puffiness.
Cypress – good for circulation and other symptoms.
Geranium – eases symptoms.
Melissa – helps nervousness.
Millepertuis – eases symptoms.
Parsley – good for fluid retention.
Rose – alleviates many symptoms.

Treatment for menopausal symptoms

This can be used as a bath essence or as a massage oil – or a bath first followed by a massage!

30ml (2 tablespoons) grapeseed oil
2 capsules evening primrose oil
1 capsule wheatgerm oil
10 drops essential oil of chamomile
5 drops essential oil of clary sage
8 drops essential oil of melissa
5 drops essential oil of rose
50ml bottle

Add ingredients to the bottle and shake well. Before use, let it rest for a couple of days in a cool, dark place. For use in the bath – pour 8 drops under running water. Alternatively, use this oil to massage the body from the ankles upwards, feet, knees and inner thighs. Clockwise around the solar plexus, nape of the neck, temples, shoulders, arms and hands. Do this once a day until symptoms ease. This oil will keep for two to three months. ❧

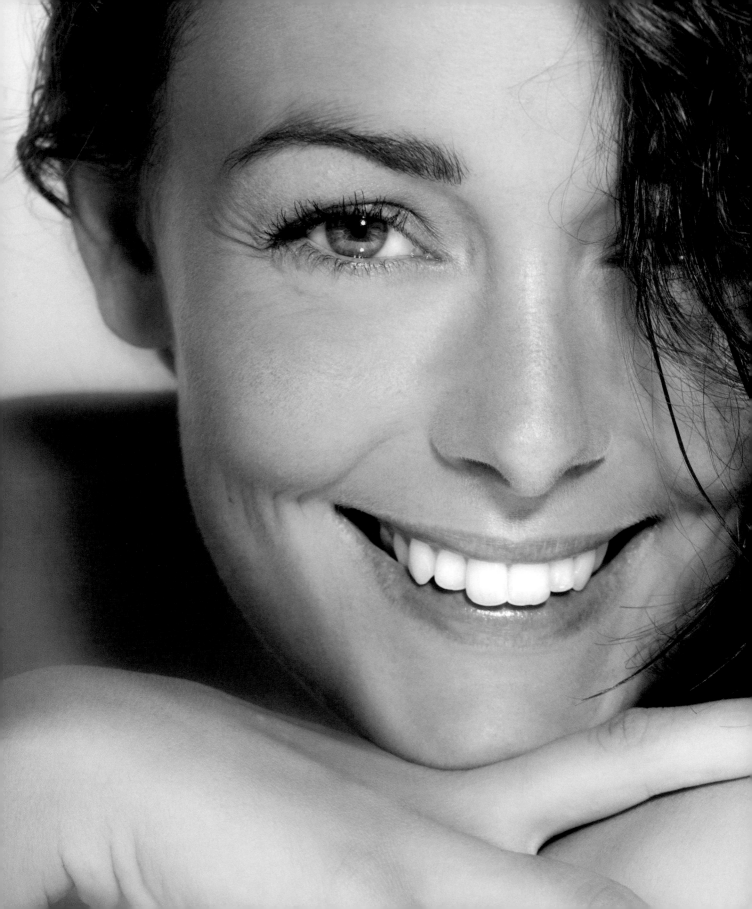

Eyes

The eyes are sometimes referred to as the window of your soul. They are wonderful tools of expression – they can smile, glare, show anger and anxiety, observe the world and cry – and can be the most beautiful facial feature. With this in mind it is so important to look after them.

Many people experience eye problems and this is not surprising when you realize what our eyes have to deal with on a daily basis. They are constantly in contact with irritants and pollutants such as dust and smoke, and even the wind can cause problems – a pair of large sunglasses will protect against all of these.

Conjunctivitis, a painful inflammatory condition, is one of the most common eye complaints. Allergies such as hay fever can also cause redness and irritation. Lack of sleep and bad lighting are also factors, as are extended periods spent at the computer. By staring at a computer screen we put an incredible amount of stress on our eyes. The screens give off radiation and as we strain to look at the print they can become sore and irritated, and some computer users complain of permanent headaches.

Make-up can also cause eye problems and allergic reactions are not uncommon. Don't use saliva to smudge eye make-up as this can provoke infections. Eye pencils and mascaras should be changed regularly and if you like to apply kohl to the inner rim of your eye, be careful. Sometimes colour can get into the eye membrane, resulting in blurred vision, itchy eyes and redness.

Add linseed capsules and wheatgerm oil to your diet and make sure you eat plenty of foods rich in vitamin A. Vitamin A is a vital nutrient because it forms part of the chemical structure of the eye's light-sensitive areas. This means that some anorexics and people with digestive complaints may experience eye problems. Try to drink a glass of carrot and celery juice every day, as it's full of vitamin A and thus good for your eyes. Eat plenty of dark green vegetables such as spinach and curly kale. Watercress and parsley are helpful too, as are pumpkins, apricots and oily fish.

Palming your eyes for a few minutes a day is also a great treatment – place the bottom of each palm over your eyes for a few minutes, pressing your palm over your eyeball and massaging slightly. This is a wonderful remedy for sore, tired eyes. **Note:** If you wear contacts remove them first!

It is very rare that people think about doing any eye exercises, but they are so helpful for strengthening the eye muscles. When I was little my grandfather and I used to go for walks and he would ask me how many different colour greens I could see. I would try to count them all – dark green trees through to light green shrubs. He would make me distinguish between all the different leaf shapes, both nearby and in the distance and then ask me to pick out flowers of different colours – a great eye strengthening exercise.

Never use pure essential oils in your eyes, as they could be very dangerous. Instead use an eyebath containing an infusion (see page 11) – both marigold and chamomile are good for this. Other good things to try are rose, fennel, cucumber and cornflower. To generally enhance the health of your eyes, and to soothe your eyes when pollen levels are high, put a few drops of essential oil of chamomile into a bowl of hot water and place nearby.

The eyes are sometimes referred to as the window of your soul ... and can be the most beautiful facial feature.

Remedies for minor eye problems

Eyebath for stressed eyes

3–4 heads of either marigold or
*   chamomile (or a dessertspoon*
*   of loose leaves)*
300ml (½ pint) water

In a small saucepan, bring the water and your chosen herb to the boil. Remove from the heat and allow it to stand in the fridge for up to three hours or, better still, overnight. Strain the mixture before use. Transfer a little to an eyebath and bathe both eyes daily when they are tired. Make up a fresh solution every time.

Sea salt eyebath for stressed eyes

Dissolve 1 tablespoon coarse sea salt in 300ml (½ pint) boiled water. When cool, transfer to an eye bath and bathe your eyes. Make up a fresh solution every time and use daily for two to three days. ❧

Cleansing eye vapour

2 heads of chamomile or 1 tea bag
600ml (1 pint) water
2 drops essential oil of chamomile

In a small saucepan, bring the water and chamomile to the boil. Remove from the heat and leave to infuse for five minutes. Transfer to a bowl and mix in the essential oil of chamomile. Cover your head with a towel and lean over the bowl for a few minutes. Open your eyes, blinking often – the soothing vapours will disinfect and soothe them. Afterwards, lie on your bed with two cold chamomile tea bags placed over your eyes. This treatment is particularly good when you have a cold or flu, but is also good for tired and irritated eyes. ❧

Hot and cold eye washes

To refresh tired eyes, try sponging cold peppermint tea around the eye area. If you'd prefer something warm try chamomile tea. ❧

Scented spray for stressed and tired eyes

Add a few drops of essential oil of chamomile, lavender or eucalyptus to a spray bottle of boiled water. Spray around you. The humidity of the spray plus the essential oils will help decongest the eyes. ❧

Rose eye treatment

This is good for tired, sore eyes, puffiness and irritation.

1 handful organic rose petals
300ml (½ pint) water

Add the rose petals to the water in a saucepan and bring to the boil for a few minutes. Let it cool and pour into a sterilized bottle (rinsed with boiling water). Use cotton wool to gently wash the solution around your eyes, morning and night. It will keep for three to four days in the fridge. ❧

Puffy eyes

We all suffer from puffy eyes occasionally. For an instant remedy, witch hazel is great. Put some in the freezer for a short while then add to some cool, boiled water (half a cup of each will suffice). Add a little to some cotton wool and apply to both eyes for a few minutes.

Green tea compress for puffy eyes

Burning the candle at both ends or strong, heavy eye creams can provoke puffiness. Chamomile tea would also work well here.

Make up some green tea as normal and let cool slightly. Pour into an ice cube tray and freeze. When needed, wrap a cube in a tissue or a piece of gauze and use as a compress, alternating between each eye. ❧

Treatment for puffy eyes

4 tablespoons oats
½ cucumber, liquidized
1 drop essential oil of rose,
*   chamomile or lavender*
Gauze

In a small saucepan, make up a porridge using the oats and a little water. Leave to cool. Mix in the liquidized cucumber and the essential oil of your choice. Spread the mixture onto a piece of gauze, folding it over into a large band. Lie down and apply to the eyes, relaxing for at least five minutes. ❧

Bags under the eyes

Late nights, too much alcohol, cigarette smoke and allergies can all cause bags. Heavy creams can also contribute and it is all too easy to fall into their trap – you think they are working when really they are causing the problem.

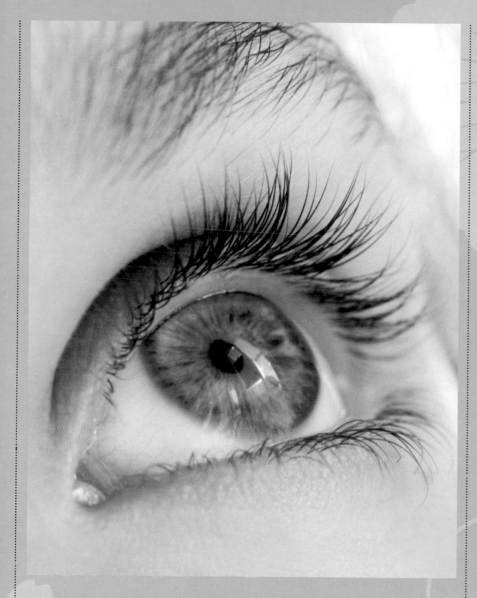

they don't grow back, so be careful. This recipe is a great conditioner.

Eyebrow shine

1 tablespoon white clay powder
5ml (1 teaspoon) jojoba oil
1 capsule wheatgerm oil
1 drop essential oil of rose

Make a paste with the white clay powder and a little warm water, and then slowly stir in the rest of the ingredients. Treat in the same way as a mask, smoothing onto the eyebrows. Relax for five to ten minutes before rinsing off with warm water. Use cotton wool to apply cold chamomile tea to finish.

Eyelashes

Mascara remover

Mix a few drops of almond oil and wheatgerm oil together. Add a little warm water and put a little on some cotton wool. Use the solution gently to remove your mascara. This will dissolve the mascara quickly as well as lubricating and conditioning your eyelashes.

Eyelash conditioner

5ml (1 teaspoon) castor oil
3/4 teaspoon jojoba oil
1 capsule wheatgerm oil
50ml bottle

Mix together in the bottle. At night, after cleansing, use your fingertips to apply to the eyelashes. This oil will make them supple and help their growth. This will keep for up to two months.

Eye gel

½ cucumber, liquidized
1 capsule wheatgerm oil
50ml herbal infusion – marigold, fennel, parsley or comfrey

Make up the infusion using a teaspoon of your chosen herb and 50ml boiled water. Let cool, strain, then stir into the cucumber with the wheatgerm capsule. Apply a little of the gel to your fingertips and pat into the area around the eye. This will boost the circulation, reduce puffiness and lines and wrinkles too. Keep in the fridge and use in the next three days.

Eyebrows

Eyebrows embellish the eyes and are important to the face but many women pluck them too much. A simple reshape is fine but sometimes

HOW TO GET A GOOD NIGHT'S SLEEP

Sleeping well can be anti-ageing for both the body and mind as it enhances the production of melatonin by the pineal gland (melatonin controls our 'body clock', regulating our sleep–wake cycle).

Sleep rejuvenates and restores, and helps increase antioxidant activities to counter the effects of free radicals (rogue unstable cells that can lead to disease; antioxidants bind with free radical cells before they can cause damage within the body). However, most people never stop to think about the good effects sleep has on our health.

Insomnia

Most people suffer from sleeplessness at some time or another and it's usually due to stress – health, money, relationships and careers are the principal worries that tend to keep us awake. They are hard to control as they prey on our minds during the night, worrying us for answers – I find it useful to keep a pen and paper beside my bed, so I can note down any thoughts and concerns, thus emptying my mind.

Lifestyle is a major contributor too. What we eat and when, or eating too fast or too late can all lead to digestive problems that will affect our sleeping patterns (cramps and wind make for an uncomfortable night). Our digestive systems slow down at night and eating late requires them to work overtime – we need to respect our body's functions.

A sedentary life, with little or no exercise or a lifestyle that involves too much exercise and not enough rest, will also contribute to insomnia. States of extreme fatigue go hand in hand with insomnia. Television before bed, especially terrible news footage, will stimulate the mind at a time when we need to relax.

There is nothing wrong with waking up for a few minutes a night as long as you go back to your dreams. As we grow older we will find that we need less sleep (good sleep) and we need to let go of the idea that we require so many hours. Older members of my family only need five or six hours of good sleep a night in order to be healthy. Their wakeful hours are used in a productive manner – writing, exercising and reading.

An herbal tisane (see page 11) before bed can really help you to relax. Good ones to try include linden tea (tilleul), verbena (vervein), chamomile, lavender, orange leaves, eucalyptus leaves, passiflora and lettuce leaves. Good tisanes to aid your digestion include basil, fennel, aniseeds, celery and coriander. But don't drink peppermint tea before bed since this acts as a stimulant.

Make sure your bedroom is well ventilated as a stuffy room could leave you feeling dehydrated and desperate for air. Open your bedroom window half-an-hour before sleep, closing it before you get into bed. In the summer it is good to sleep with the window open (unless your room backs on to a road with heavy traffic). Invest in a window box and plant it with lavender in the summer. In the winter bring orange, lemon or mandarin trees inside and you will notice the beneficial effects of their wonderful smell instantly.

Essential oils will help you to enjoy a good sleep. They can be relaxing, calming, de-stressing and slightly hypnotic, easy to use and have wonderful scents too.

Good sleep-inducing essential oils are: chamomile, lavender, bergamot, orange, neroli, melissa and clary sage.

Remedies for a good night's sleep

Relaxing room vaporizer

A few squirts of this spray in your bedroom an hour before bedtime will help promote a good sleep.

50ml lavender infusion
5 drops essential oil of sandalwood

5 drops essential oil of bergamot
5 drops essential oil of chamomile
2 drops essential oil of neroli
2 drops essential oil of lavender
50ml spray bottle

Put three to four sprigs of lavender into a saucepan and cover with 600ml (1 pint) water. Bring to the boil then leave to infuse for twenty minutes. Strain and pour 50ml into the bottle. Add the essential oils. Shake well before use. This will keep for ten days in a cool place. ❧

Room vaporizer to relieve snoring

If you have a cold or if you snore or have breathing difficulties this spray will help you. Spray it around your bedroom an hour before bedtime, alternatively you could spray a little on a tissue and place on your bedside table.

100ml cooled down boiled water
5 drops essential oil of eucalyptus
5 drops essential oil of chamomile
2 drops essential oil of peppermint
5 drops essential oil of frankincense or hyssop
2 drops essential oil of lavender
100ml bottle

Pour ingredients into the bottle and shake well. This will keep for ten days in a cool place. ❧

Relaxing room fragrance

This is a formulation that I like a lot. Place a few drops on a tissue and leave beside your bed. When you sleep you will inhale the fumes

gently – they will help you calm down, relax and sleep. It is so useful particularly because you can take it with you when you travel.

5ml (1 teaspoon) grapeseed oil
1 capsule wheatgerm oil
5 drops essential oil of neroli
10 drops essential oil of lavender
5 drops essential oil of chamomile
10 drops essential oil of either bergamot or petit grain
10 drops essential oil of melissa
10ml bottle with a dropper

Pour ingredients into the bottle and shake well. Apply a couple of drops on a tissue and leave by your bed or put it into your pyjama pocket. (Small bottles with droppers can be obtained from a chemist or pharmacy.) ❧

Scented bed linen

When you wash your bed linen, add a few drops of essential oil of lavender to the conditioner compartment of your washing machine. Alternatively, put a few drops on a flannel and place it with the rest of your washing in the drum of your tumble dryer.

You can also scent the sheets in the cupboard – insert tissues impregnated with essential oil of lavender, orange or melissa in between the bed linen.

Relaxing pot pourri

Bring a bowl of dried lavender flowers, melissa, orange leaves and roses into your bedroom. Leave near your bed.

Massage before bedtime

A massage a few hours before bed will also help you to relax.

15ml (1 tablespoon) almond oil
1 drop essential oil of melissa
2 drops essential oil of frankincense
1 drop essential oil of basil
2 drops essential oil of lavender, orange, petit grain or neroli

Add the drops of essential oil to the almond oil. Begin with the feet, massaging the oil in gently. Then do one leg at a time, working the oil into your knees and up the thighs. Rub into the bottom and the hips and the lower part of your back. Then massage into the nape of the neck and gently around the temples and the sinus area. Finish by massaging the oil into the chest area and work clockwise around the solar plexus. Use long, slow movements, breathe deeply and relax. Lie down for a few moments with a cushion under your feet. ❧

Mouth

The mouth is one of the hardest working parts of the body. It is through the mouth that most substances are introduced to our body – we use it to eat, drink, talk – and breathe.

Good digestion begins in the mouth and our teeth are the key. They help us break down our food into easily digestible matter, yet many of us do not know how to chew. Chewing not only encourages a good flow of saliva (required for digestion), but also exercises the jawbone and facial muscles, improving circulation and helping to keep a youthful look. By taking more time to chew, we will eat less – good news for dieters!

Teeth and gums

According to my dentist, gum disease is the greatest cause of tooth loss and plaque is the main problem. These tiny bacteria produce irritating enzymes that result in inflammation and gingivitis. If left to harden they turn into tartar, a hard deposit that can lead to gum disease. The good news is that this unattractive disease can be easily avoided.

A confident, white smile is envied by most of us but there is more to looking after your teeth than just brushing them twice a day. A balanced diet is necessary for good teeth and gum health, and it is important to try to avoid sugar. Make sure you change your toothbrush every six weeks. Clean it regularly – dissolve a little bicarbonate of soda in some water and submerge the brush for a few minutes. Don't brush your teeth too hard and floss before brushing. Beware of abrasive toothpastes. Above all visit your dentist regularly.

Sage tooth whitener

Sage is a wonderful old herbal remedy for cleaning teeth. You can simply chew sage leaves or try making this natural whitener. It's great for removing coffee and tobacco stains.

2 tablespoons coarse sea salt
1 large tablespoon fresh culinary sage
2 mint leaves
Jar

Blend ingredients to a fine consistency with a pestle and mortar. Put into a glass jar, dipping toothbrush into the mixture when needed. Brush teeth with it twice a day. Although it is salty, try and keep the mixture in the mouth for at least a minute. Rinse. This will make enough for approximately a week. ༅

Angelica mouthwash

Promotes healthy gums and fresh breath.

60g angelica stems (buy from a Chinese herbalist or health food shop)
½ litre vodka
1 litre still mineral water
6 cloves
2-litre bottle

Mix together in the bottle then leave in the dark for two weeks. When required, dilute a capful in a glass of warm water and use as a mouthwash. ༅

Peppermint cure for toothache/sore gums

Add a drop of essential oil of peppermint to some cotton wool and place inside the mouth on the affected area. Clove oil also works well. ༅

Sage oil for gum infections

20ml (2 dessert spoons) sesame oil
2 tablespoons fresh culinary sage
2 pinches coarse sea salt
Jar

Blend the mixture until fine and put into a glass jar. Dip your finger into the mixture and massage your gums with it twice a day. Try and keep in your mouth for as long as possible. Rinse with warm water and follow with the appropriate mouthwash. This will make enough for two days. ༅

Mouthwash for bleeding gums

1 handful rose petals
600ml (1 pint) water
1 drop essential oil of rose
150ml water
½-litre bottle

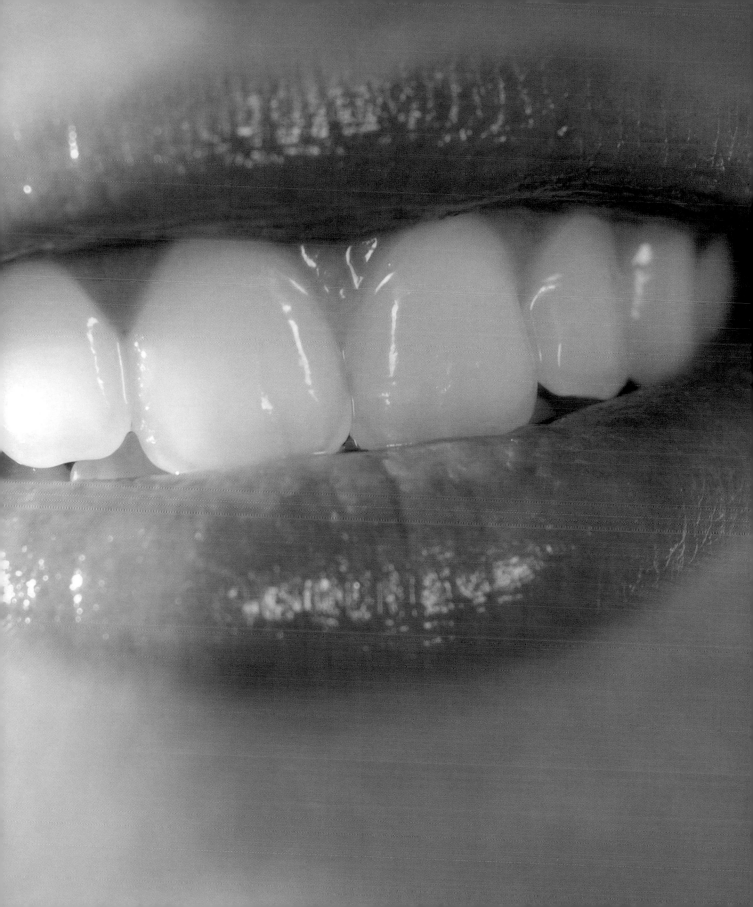

Make a rose petal infusion – cover the rose petals with the 600ml (1 pint) of water, bring to the boil. Leave to cool and infuse for half-an-hour. Strain. Add 200ml of the infusion to 150ml water containing a drop of essential oil of rose. Stir. Gargle for a few moments, keep in the mouth before spitting out and repeating. Repeat two to three times a day. Consult your dentist if symptoms persist. ❧

Gum cleanser oil

This oil is good for tooth enamel. It is also a gentle whitener and the sesame oil is wonderful for removing unwanted bacteria. Make sure you don't swallow it though!

20ml (2 dessert spoons) sesame oil
10ml (1 dessert spoon) strong
  peppermint tea, cooled
1 capsule wheatgerm oil
50ml bottle

Mix ingredients together and pour into the bottle. To use, pour a little oil into a cup and dip your index finger into it. Massage into the gums in circular movements. Keep in mouth for a few minutes before rinsing with warm water. Use twice a day for a couple of days. Will keep for up to two months. ❧

Spicy mouthwash for bad breath

Bad breath or halitosis can become persistent and may indicate decayed teeth or a gum infection. Chew coriander, fennel, anise, caraway or cardamom seeds – these all contain cleansing essential oils. Cloves and cinnamon also have a breath-freshening action. Drink carrot, celery and apple juices for the digestion. Nettle tea is also good. The spicy mouthwash described below will also help.

1 stick cinnamon or 1 tablespoon
  ground cinnamon
1/2 tablespoon grated nutmeg
5 cloves
1/2 tablespoon aniseeds
100ml vodka
150ml nettle or peppermint tea
5 drops essential oil of peppermint
600ml (1 pint) water
1-litre bottle

Mix ingredients together, pour into the bottle and leave in a dark place for a week. Shake before use. Dilute a tablespoon of the mouthwash in a glass of water and gargle every morning. Keeps for up to two months. ❧

Liquorice mouthwash for fresh breath

2 sticks liquorice
300ml (1/2 pint) water
1 slice fresh ginger
1 drop essential oil of ginger,
  cardamom or fennel
1/2-litre bottle

In a small saucepan, bring the liquorice and water to the boil. Remove from the heat and add the fresh ginger. Leave to infuse for twenty minutes; then spoon out the liquorice and ginger. Pour into a bottle and add your oil. Shake well before use. Dilute a capful in a glass of water and use twice a day after brushing. Will keep for five days in the fridge. ❧

Mouth ulcers

Mouth ulcers can be caused by acidity or can occur when you are feeling run down. Mouth ulcers react to many foods. Avoid eating acidic foods such as citrus fruits, although strangely, a few drops of fresh lemon juice applied to the ulcer will have an antiseptic, astringent effect (be warned though – it does hurt a little). Wheatgerm and lecithin capsules can help, as can flax oil – drizzle it over vegetables or take a tablespoon in the morning with a glass of warm water. It will help soothe inflammation and promote healing.

Soothing tisanes made from the fresh leaves of nettle, peppermint and watercress can help, so can milky alkaline foods (if you have an intolerance try soya or rice milk). Oily fish and seaweeds are also good.

Lips

Recent research in the US suggests that some pigments contained in shop-bought lipsticks are potentially unsafe. Many include petroleum-derived chemicals. These cover the lips in a film, trapping much-needed moisture on the surface. Lips become accustomed to it and the product will need to be applied constantly.

The lips only have three to five layers of skin compared with fifteen on the rest of the body. They are lucky enough to have a small amount of melanin to protect them from the sun's harmful rays, but even then, the sun combined with chemical lipsticks and balms mean they can still be susceptible to skin cancer.

Lip plump

We are constantly looking for new ways of enhancing our lips – from collagen injections to high-street lip plumps. I prefer to use a natural balm. Massage it into your lips twice a day and you will have a fuller pout in no time.

10ml (1 dessert spoon) jojoba oil
5ml (1 teaspoon) castor oil
5ml (1 teaspoon) argan oil
2 capsules wheatgerm oil
50ml bottle

Mix the ingredients together in the bottle and apply to the lips, gently pressing in the oil with the fingertips. Massage into the skin around the mouth in a clockwise direction, pulling out both the upper and lower lips slightly and rubbing in. Apply a little more oil to the lips and leave for a few minutes before removing the surplus with a tissue. Ideally use twice a day. Keeps for a month in the fridge. ᴥ

Lip protector

This is excellent for chapped lips!

5ml (1 teaspoon) jojoba oil
2 tablespoons Manuka honey
5ml (1 teaspoon) lavender flower
   water (from a decoction)
½ drop essential oil of peppermint
1 drop essential oil of lemon

Mix the ingredients together and apply as needed (To get ½ drop of peppermint oil put a drop in a teaspoon and use half.) Massage gently into the lips before applying lipstick or make-up. ᴥ

Protective lip gloss for chapped lips

Carrot essential oil is especially good here but you can alternate between geranium, palmarosa, lemon and rose.

25g organic beeswax
15ml (1 tablespoon) avocado oil
15ml (1 tablespoon) castor oil
5ml (1 teaspoon) jojoba oil
1 capsule evening primrose oil
2 capsules wheatgerm oil
6 drops essential oil of carrot

Melt the beeswax using the bain-marie method (see page 12), then add the avocado and castor oils, stirring all the time. Add the jojoba oil, and the oil from the evening primrose and wheatgerm capsules. Remove from the heat and let cool slightly. Add the essential oil of carrot before transferring into two small jars – one for the home and one for your handbag! This will keep for two to three months, stored in the fridge. ᴥ

Lip stain

I've used cherries in this recipe but try experimenting with elderberries, blackcurrants or even beetroot!

450g (1lb) dark cherries
600ml (1 pint) water
5ml (1 teaspoon) castor oil

10ml (1 dessert spoon) jojoba oil
10g organic beeswax
2 tablespoons Manuka honey
1 capsule wheatgerm oil
Jar

Cover the cherries in the water and bring to the boil in a large saucepan. Simmer until the liquid has reduced to a third. Strain to remove stones and reserve the juice. In a bain-marie, melt the beeswax, jojoba and castor oil gently. Add the Manuka honey and wheatgerm oil. Slowly stir in a dessertspoon of the cherry juice and leave to cool a little. Transfer to a small jar. This will keep in the fridge for over a month. Apply with finger or lip brush. ᴥ

Cold sore remedy

Cold sores often appear at the most inconvenient times but this remedy will help.

5ml (1 teaspoon) castor oil
5ml (1 teaspoon) sesame oil
1 capsule wheatgerm oil
2 drops essential oil of geranium
2 drops essential oil of chamomile
1 drop essential oil of tea tree
1 drop essential oil of lavender
1 drop essential oil of rose
A few drops freshly squeezed lemon
   juice
150ml boiled water, cooled
½-litre bottle

Pour the ingredients into a bottle. Use a cotton bud to apply the oil to the cold sore two to three times a day. This will keep for two weeks in the fridge. ᴥ

BOOSTING THE IMMUNE SYSTEM

Happiness is a great way to boost your immune system to better enable you to face the many viruses that flourish during the winter months.

Biological science is still beginning to understand the mysteries of life energies. For the body to be protected and rejuvenated, it will depend on being able to activate and have access to the energies that support our life force. It is our life force that nourishes us, controls our growth, detoxifies and rejuvenates at all times, regenerating our cells.

All living things are supported by this life force and it is in all of us, from flowers to animals to humans. Traditional medicinal practices such as ayurveda and various Chinese therapies all work with this energy. By eating the right food you can reinforce this energy and, in turn, boost your immune system.

The Swiss physician Bircher-Benner prescribed a diet of fruit, vegetables and nuts in order to heal his patients at his sanatorium. Marguerite Maury reinforced this by noting the importance of essential oils to our health – protecting us from diseases, boosting our immune systems, creating a dynamic harmony between the mind and body and giving us back our lost energy.

The human body requires constant loving and tender care to fight and defend us against viruses. Vitamins A, B, C and D are all essential, as is protein. Vitamins A and B are particularly relevant to the immune system. Vitamin A maintains the health of the respiratory passages and people who are deficient in it increase their susceptibility to infections. Eat liver, watercress and apricots. Recent research has also shown a correlation between vitamin B deficiency and lung disease. Eat lots of green leafy vegetables, Marmite and brewer's yeast. Also include in your diet: almonds, cucumber, dates, green beans and oats.

Raw fruits and vegetables (high in vitamin C) also contain a small percentage of essential oils and they will help to eliminate and detoxify. By eating these and using essential oils at the same time, you can help build up resistance to infections.

Boosting the immune system with essential oils

Good immune boosting essential oils include: rosemary, marjoram, melissa, eucalyptus, ravensare, cajuput, angelica, tea tree, lavender, ginger, peppermint, lemon, grapefruit, thyme and ylang-ylang.

Immune boosting flower water

This has great bactericide properties and helps fight infections.

100ml warm, boiled water
3 drops essential oil of rosemary
2 drops essential oil of eucalyptus
3 drops essential oil of melissa
4 drops essential oil of grapefruit
100ml spray bottle

Fill the bottle with the water and add the essential oils. Shake well. Spray your home or workspace a few times a day. This will keep for two weeks in a cool place. ❧

Inhalation to boost the immune system

Place a bowl of water in your place of work and add five drops of essential oil chosen from the list above. Combine two oils, two drops of one and three of the other. ❧

Inhalation for colds and fevers

If you have been shivering or feel a fever coming on, an inhalation is good. Add one drop of essential oil of eucalyptus or tea tree and one drop of essential oil of ravensare to a bowl of boiling water. Place a towel over your head and inhale the fumes for at least five minutes. Follow with a massage with the antiseptic oil described on page 111. ❧

Antiseptic gargle for sore throats

Sore throats can be extremely painful and it is best to avoid hard foods like bread and crisps. Hot spices can also hurt and remember not to smoke!

300ml (½ pint) boiled water
Freshly squeezed juice of half a lemon
1 dessertspoon Manuka honey
1 drop essential oil of either rose or
    geranium

Add the ingredients to a large glass and use as a gargle three to five times a day until symptoms are reduced.

Alternatively, make an infusion of either rose petals or eucalyptus leaves (a handful of each) – add to 600ml (1 pint) of water and bring to the boil. Leave to cool, then strain. For the gargle, add the lemon and honey to one-quarter of the solution. Use as before. ❧

Frozen lemon and pineapple sore throat remedy

Freshly squeezed juice of 2 lemons
300ml (½ pint) pineapple juice
1 tablespoon Manuka honey

Mix the ingredients together and pour into an ice cube tray. Freeze. Suck on individual cubes to relieve a sore throat. ❧

Antiseptic massage oil
This is good for helping to prevent colds and flu.

10ml (1 dessert spoon) grapeseed oil
1 capsule wheatgerm oil
2 drops essential oil of marjoram,
    niaouli or cajuput
2 drops essential oil of eucalyptus

Mix ingredients together and gently massage the oil into the sinus area,

temples, nape of neck, torso and forehead. Repeat a few times during the day. ❧

Bath for aches and pains
A bad bout of flu can result in aching joints and muscles but this bath will help.

2 drops essential oil of tea tree
2 drops essential oil of eucalyptus
2 drops essential oil of pine

Add the oils to a warm bath and relax for fifteen minutes. ❧

Mustard bath
Mustard is great for colds and flu; it will soothe aching limbs and relieve chills. It will make you sweat but remember it is relieving toxins!

1 tablespoon powdered mustard
2 drops essential oil of eucalyptus,
    niaouli or cajuput
2 drops essential oil of ravensare
2 drops essential oil of rosemary
2 drops essential oil of pine

Mix the mustard powder with a little water to make a paste. Stir in the essential oils and disperse in the bath. Relax. ❧

Barrier oil
This oil protects against infections and a bottle can be kept in your pocket and taken with you on public transport.

10ml (1 dessert spoon) grapeseed oil
1 capsule wheatgerm oil

2 drops essential oil of geranium,
    rose or clove
2 drops essential oil of peppermint
2 drops essential oil of rosemary
    or thyme
50ml bottle

Mix ingredients together in the bottle and use to rub under and inside nose and sinus area. Put a few drops on a tissue and inhale when needed. It acts as a barrier against germs. It will keep for two to three months. ❧

Body oil
Essential oils also work with external application and their natural antibiotic and antiseptic properties will penetrate the skin and enter the respiratory system through inhalation.

Good antibiotic and antiseptic oils to try are: eucalyptus, ravensare, melissa, marjoram, thyme, clove, pine and cypress.

Choose three different oils from this list to make the following body oil, five drops of each. This is a great preventative against colds and flu.

25ml (2½ dessert spoons) almond oil
25ml (2½ dessert spoons) soya oil
1 capsule wheatgerm oil
1 capsule evening primrose oil
3 essential oils from the above list,
    5 drops of each
50ml bottle

Mix ingredients together and massage over body, starting with the limbs and ending with the chest area. Use daily for a week. The oil will keep for two to three months. ❧

Jawline and neck

The jawline and neck area is very delicate and will certainly need attention sooner rather than later as it is one of the first places to show your age. When moisturizing your face, always remember to take some of the cream or oil down over your jawline to your neck. Wrinkles will appear as the skin loses its elasticity and a double chin could become a permanent feature!

But help is at hand – essential oils can work wonders, as can massage, exercise and ensuring you have good posture – so there is no need to panic.

Jawline and neck massage

First cleanse your face and neck, relaxing and letting go of any tension. Place your fingers under your cheekbones and massage, gently lifting and holding for a count of five. These movements will come naturally as you breathe in and out. Release and count to five again. Massage the jawline in the same way – gently lifting, pinching and holding the skin. Follow the line of the jaw to the ears.

Support the back of the neck with one hand, lifting and stretching

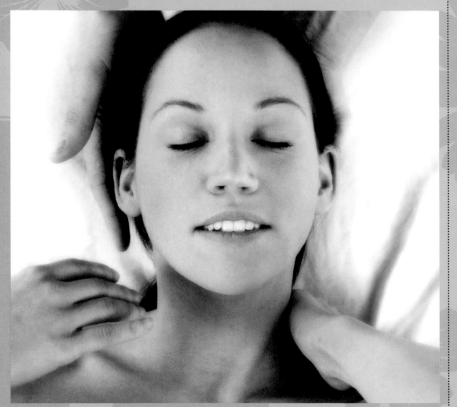

gently and pulling slightly. Do the same with the other hand, repeating a few times. Find the pressure points (on either side) at the base of your skull and massage. All the tension will be released and any headaches will disappear. Sit up straight in your chair, then lean forward in your seat. Finish by using both hands to pull the skin on either side of the neck gently, starting at the base and working to the top.

Treatments for the neck

Sandalwood neck oil

10ml (1 dessert spoon) jojoba oil
8ml (1½ teaspoons) avocado oil
2 capsules borage oil
4 capsules wheatgerm oil
10 drops essential oil of sandalwood
5 drops essential oil of bois de rose
2 drops essential oil of either petit grain or orange
50ml bottle

Mix together in the bottle and shake well. To help penetration of the oil, place a hot flannel on your face for a few minutes. Apply every night until used up – this recipe gives enough for two to three weeks' supply. Keep it in the fridge or a cool place. Do this two or three times a year. ♫

Mild exfoliator

Use this to gently exfoliate the neck before you apply the moisturizing oil, below. The amounts given below make enough for one application.

1 teaspoon sunflower seeds, ground
6 almonds, crushed
½ fresh papaya, peeled and blended
5ml (1 teaspoon) avocado oil
1 capsule wheatgerm oil

Mix all the ingredients together and apply to your neck and décolleté. Massage in using circular movements. Leave on for a few minutes then rinse with warm water. Do twice a month.

Moisturizing neck oil

Rose, palmarosa, galbanum, vetiver, black pepper, sandalwood and orange are all great essential oils to use. You need three essential oils in total, three drops of each, so alternate between them according to your preference.

10ml (1 dessert spoon) borage oil
10ml (1 dessert spoon) castor oil
10ml (1 dessert spoon) argan oil
20ml (2 dessert spoons) jojoba oil
30ml (2 tablespoons) almond oil
1 capsule evening primrose oil
2 capsules wheatgerm oil
3 drops essential oil of rose
3 drops essential oil of galbanum
3 drops essential oil of orange
100ml bottle

Mix together in the bottle and shake well. Massage it in to your neck once a day, preferably at night. This oil will keep for approximately one month in the fridge or in a cool place away from light.

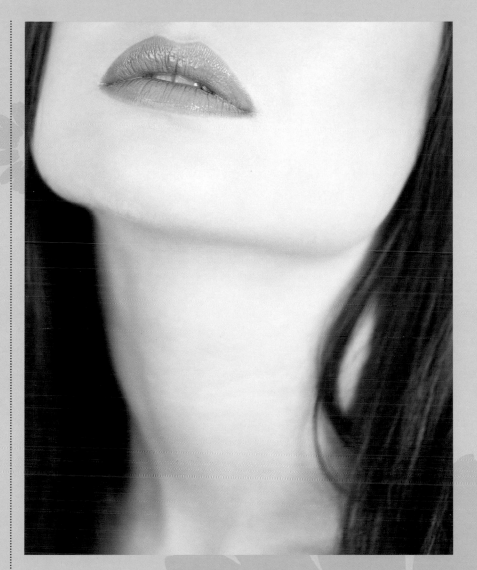

Firming neck mask

I've used rose and sandalwood essential oils here but you can swap between the oils listed above for the moisturizing neck oil. The amounts given here should be enough for three applications. The mask will keep in the fridge for approximately two weeks.

1 tablespoon white clay powder
10ml (1 dessert spoon) rosewater
1 capsule wheatgerm oil

30ml (2 tablespoons) aloe vera juice,
  organic if possible
1 drop essential oil of rose
1 drop essential oil of sandalwood

Slowly mix together the clay, rosewater, wheatgerm oil and aloe vera juice to form a paste. Make sure there are no lumps. Stir in the essential oils. Apply to the neck and leave on for five minutes before rinsing off with warm water.

Breasts

The breasts contain no muscle, only fat cells, glands and milk ducts surrounded by connective tissue. Consequently, it is hard to keep breasts firm and upright – with age they start to sag and the supporting muscles become stretched and slack.

The size and shape of the breasts is determined by their fatty adipose tissue. Gaining or losing weight, hormonal changes and pregnancy can all produce changes in breast shape. Not all these changes are welcome, however, and as a result many women turn to implants and reductions.

Slack pectoral muscles that haven't been exercised can cause the breasts to sag. These muscles are located in the chest, behind the breast tissue, upper arms and back. Swimming, especially breaststroke, and push-ups are two of the best activities for strengthening and toning these supporting muscles, and lifting and firming the bust line. With regular exercise, women with heavy breasts will gain a better shape and sleeker appearance, with firmer contours. Those with smaller breasts will develop a more firm, prominent shape.

Essential oils, with their natural plant hormones and astringent properties can really help firm and tone the pectoral muscles.

Treatments for firmer breasts

Aromatic vinegar lotion

This lotion is great for firming the connective tissue around the breasts. It is easy to make – just add some fresh or dried herbs to a bottle of cider or white wine vinegar. Good herbs to use are mint, basil, lavender, rosemary and thyme. You can also use essential oils if you prefer – bois de rose, rose, peppermint, ylang-ylang and lavender all work well.

6–10 tablespoons dried herbs or a handful of fresh herbs or 15 drops of one of the essential oils listed above
1/2 litre cider or white wine vinegar
3/4 litre boiled cold water
2-litre bottle

Add your chosen herb or essential oil to the bottle of vinegar. Keep in the dark for approximately two weeks. Add the water. Use cotton wool to apply the lotion in circular movements to each breast. Do this a few times. Let dry. Try using this preparation for two months. ❧

Firming ice cubes

This is an old remedy for firming the breasts as favoured by French belles.

300ml (1/2 pint) water
1 handful fresh parsley
100ml aloe vera juice
5 drops essential oil of cypress
5 drops essential oil of rose

Boil the water and pour over the parsley. Leave to infuse for 20 minutes. Stir in the aloe vera juice and the essential oils. Mix well. Pour into an ice cube tray and leave to cool before transferring to the freezer. After a shower or a bath rub a cube around the breast. Dry with a soft towel. ❧

Breasts and pregnancy

For nine months the hormones have been priming the glands for milk production so the breasts are heavy and full. Breastfeeding should be a joy to the mother as it is the time that the bond between her and her baby becomes even stronger. Many women, though, are misinformed and believe that their breasts will sag and lose their firmness. In fact, the baby's suckling action actually tones up the muscles!

Breastfeeding has so many wonderful advantages. During the first few days after birth the breasts produce a special kind of milk called colostrum that is vital for the baby's strength and overall health. Research has shown that it builds up the baby's resistance to infections. Babies who are given powdered milk from birth often have difficulties adapting to formula, which can result in colic, diarrhoea and vomiting.

To stimulate a good flow of milk add to your diet: fennel, carrots, organic honey, soya milk, beans and tofu, and wheatgerm. Eat lots of parsley – sprinkle it on brown rice, pasta, meat and vegetables. Parsley and peppermint tea is excellent too – in a pint of boiling water, infuse a tablespoon of chopped parsley with a few mint leaves. Leave for five minutes and drink. **Note:** Do not use essential oil of parsley during pregnancy as it can be very harmful.

Oil to prevent sore nipples
Many women suffer from sore and cracked nipples during breastfeeding and this can make the experience very painful. For a couple of months before the baby is due, prepare your nipples with this oil.

10ml (1 dessert spoon) jojoba or almond oil
4 capsules wheatgerm oil
A few drops freshly squeezed lemon or lime juice
50ml bottle

Mix oils together in the bottle. Add a few drops of lemon or lime juice and shake well. Apply to the tip of each nipple, massaging and pulling them for a few minutes every day. ॐ

Oil for sagging breasts
Use this oil to avoid sagging and regain firmness in breasts. Don't use until the baby has finished breast-feeding.

30ml (2 tablespoons) almond or jojoba oil
2 capsules wheatgerm oil
1 capsule evening primrose oil
1 capsule borage oil
4 drops essential oil of rose
2 drops essential oil of lemon
2 drops essential oil of lavender
1 drop essential oil of either peppermint or black pepper
50ml bottle

Mix together in the bottle and shake well. Use this oil once a day to massage the breasts and nipples. This oil will keep for up to two months. ॐ

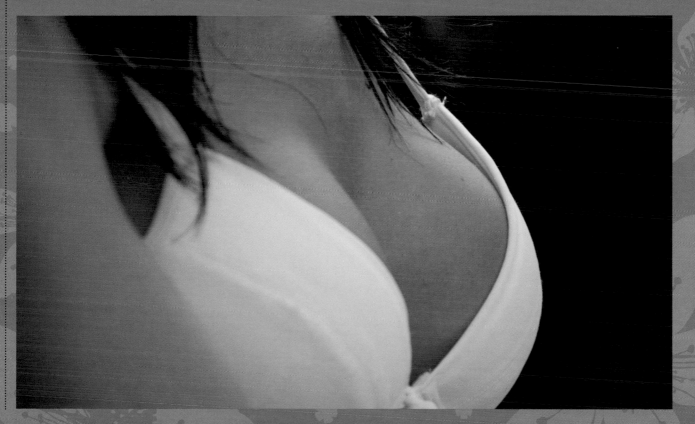

CARING FOR YOURSELF IN PREGNANCY

The nine months of a pregnancy can be among the happiest of your life, bringing strong feelings of fulfilment and love.

And it's no wonder – preparations for pregnancy start as early as puberty as a women's body awaits the event of a birth.

Pregnancy is a time of change. You will need to reconsider your lifestyle as your life will alter considerably when your bundle of joy arrives. This is a great time to remove yourself from stress and surround yourself with positive energy – flowers and plants will have an immediate effect on this, so a walk in your local park will have huge benefits. Many women embrace this change and feel a great urge to move house or redecorate!

It is important to be in good health during pregnancy as both your physical and emotional states will have a great bearing on your child's development. From conception to the first eight to ten weeks the foetus grows at an incredible rate. Taking care of your health from the very beginning is imperative if you want a healthy baby.

Remember that everything you eat and everything you apply to your skin will filter through to the foetus. The foetal cells need a plentiful supply of vitamins, minerals, amino acids and fatty acids to help growth. The nutrients you ingest will go to the foetus before your body has a chance of absorbing them. If you don't look after yourself and eat sensibly you will start to feel tired, bad tempered and stressed.

Poisons are easily passed from the mother to the baby so avoid hair dyes. These are full of chemicals and can travel through your system to the baby. Aluminium pans are another no-no and make sure you filter your tap water in case it contains lead (this has been linked to learning difficulties and can poison the nervous system). Wearing strong perfume can make you feel nauseous so change to a gentle essential oil in an oil base (for advice on which oils are safe to use in pregnancy, see page 119). You must (and this is a definite must) give up smoking during pregnancy, or even better give it up before conception. Try to avoid smoky areas too and avoid inhaling traffic fumes – cover your nose with a scarf in busy traffic.

Drink freshly squeezed juices diluted with filtered or mineral water, and herbal tisanes (see page 11) of chamomile, thyme, rosehip or sage. Use Manuka or an organic honey to sweeten them. Eat organic food if possible and enjoy the food you eat. Foods rich in magnesium help reduce anxiety and insomnia, so eat plenty of avocados and almonds – these are great as snacks too. Learn to eat slowly. A good habit to get into is taking a nap in the afternoon. Just twenty to thirty minutes of relaxation will make all the difference. Lie on your bed with your feet up – put a cushion under your knees. Make sure the nape of your neck is supported and put on some relaxing music.

Pregnancy is characterized by an upsurge in the production of oestrogen and progesterone. Such hormonal changes can bring about other changes in your system and you may experience cravings for certain foods. I remember craving sweet things like honey and marmalade and absolutely couldn't be in a room with the smell of bacon – I felt terribly nauseous and was often sick as a result! (Incidentally, this shows you how strongly smells can affect you at this time.) Other discomforts may include swellings, circulation problems, backache, insomnia and sometimes nervousness in the late stages.

Essential oils are a wonderful way of treating the many problems that appear at this time. However, they must be used very carefully. Certain oils may make you feel nauseous but others can have more serious consequences and I do not advise you to use them. The remedies here have been specially devised to include gentle essential oils in balanced proportions so your baby will benefit too. Your skin will be more sensitive during pregnancy though so you *must* do a skin patch test first (see page 8).

Good essential oils to try during pregnancy are:

Orange, lemon, mandarin, petit grain, neroli and grapefruit.

Use only a very small quantity (a couple of drops) in your bath, as a room spray or in massage – you do not want to develop an allergic reaction.

Morning sickness

Morning sickness can occur at the beginning of the pregnancy and usually wears off after a while (although some women experience it for the full nine months). Avoid strong tea or coffee, alcohol, spices, black and white pepper, and oily foods. Ginger tea with lemon and Manuka honey is extremely good for morning sickness, as is grated ginger added to your cooking. I suggest you make a ginger drink – add slices of fresh ginger to a teapot, cover with boiling water, add half a squeezed orange and half a squeezed lemon. Leave to infuse for fifteen minutes and drink throughout the day. You could also add a few drops of ginger or grapefruit essential oil to a bowl of boiling water and place it beside you when you're feeling sick. Alternatively, put a drop of pure ginger or grapefruit essential oil on a tissue and inhale when feeling nauseous (if you find ginger makes the sickness worse, use grapefruit and vice versa.)

Bad digestion/ heartburn

Too much acid in the stomach can be extremely uncomfortable, causing bloating and pain (if you feel really bad you must consult your doctor). If you are a sufferer, take chamomile, rose petals, ginger or aniseed tea with meals. I found eating small snacks helped, as did chewing slowly. You could also try adding certain herbs to your cooking – tarragon, caraway, coriander and fennel all work well. Rice or vegetables that have been cooked in aniseed tea also help, as does drinking slippery elm. (This is available in powdered form from health food shops and can be mixed to make a healthy, nutritious drink.)

Circulation problems

During pregnancy your legs will take the strain and the extra pressure can have painful consequences – swollen ankles and varicose veins are commonplace. The expanding womb constricts the blood flow to the limbs and the extra weight you are carrying makes it harder for the blood to return from the extremities to the heart.

Don't stand up for long periods and stay away from your high heels. Always raise your legs when relaxing in front of the television or reading. Keep baths at body temperature. Foods containing bioflavonoids (broccoli, citrus fruits, root vegetables and dark chocolate) will help to strengthen the blood vessels and reduce inflammation.

Constipation afflicts many pregnant women and can also have a bad effect on the circulatory system. Avoid this by eating whole grain organic muesli, oats and wheatgerm. A teaspoon of linseeds (flaxseeds) added to your breakfast cereal will have a lubricating effect on your digestion.

Massage oil for varicose veins and bad circulation

Lemon is great for circulation problems and will detoxify, encourage the circulation and strengthen the capillary walls. Cypress will encourage blood circulation and will have an astringent effect on the capillaries and veins. Orange will also calm you down and soothe your mind.

30ml (2 tablespoons) almond oil
30ml (2 tablespoons) grapeseed oil
2 capsules either wheatgerm or
*   evening primrose oil*
2 drops essential oil of cypress or
*   3 drops of petit grain*
3 drops essential oil of orange
4 drops essential oil of lemon
100ml bottle

Mix ingredients together in the bottle and shake well. Massage gently into the legs in upward strokes. Start at the ankle and work towards the thigh. Use twice a week. The oil will keep for two to three months. ❧

Footbaths

I used to collect pebbles from the beach and place them in a bowl of warm water containing a couple of drops of essential oil of lemon and one of cypress or pine. I loved rubbing my feet against the pebbles. It was so effective and great for the circulation.

A massage oil to uplift your spirit
The oils used here have uplifting qualities and will help you relax after a tiring day contending with swollen ankles and backache. Use as needed.

50ml almond oil
2 capsules wheatgerm oil
1 capsule evening primrose oil
5 drops essential oil of neroli
1 drop essential oil of lemon
4 drops essential oil of grapefruit or lemongrass
100ml bottle

Mix all the oils together well before gently massaging your lower back. (You may want to get someone to help you here, as it can be difficult!) Massage the oil into your feet, legs and ankles. Alternatively you could add three to five drops of this oil to a warm bath and relax for fifteen minutes. This oil will keep for two to three months. ꙮ

Stretchmarks
Stretchmarks often appear on the breasts, stomach, hips, thighs and bottom during and after pregnancy. The overlying skin and supporting muscles are stretched to their limit, the fibres in the deep layers tear and irregular red, white or grey 'stretch' marks appear on the surface. You'll be pleased to know that these unsightly marks can be avoided and/or their appearance reduced.

Used twice a week, this gentle mixture of essential oils will help combat them.

30ml (2 tablespoons) avocado oil
5 capsules wheatgerm oil
20 drops borage oil
10 drops argan oil
2 drops essential oil of orange
2 drops essential oil of Roman chamomile
2 drops essential oil of bois de rose
50ml bottle

Mix ingredients together and shake well. Keep for a few days in a cold place before first use. Massage the areas where you think stretchmarks might appear. This oil will keep for two to three months. ꙮ

Relaxation
Relaxing teas to aid sleep
Chamomile, linden (tilleul or lime blossom), orange leaves and lettuce leaves all induce sleep and will help to soothe emotions and make you feel calm.

Relaxing room spray
Fill a spray bottle with mineral water and add three drops essential oil of lavender, three drops essential oil of chamomile and three drops essential oil of neroli or rose. Shake bottle well and use to spray your bedroom an hour before rest. ꙮ

Massage
It is worth noting that it is not advisable to have strong back massage during pregnancy. If you

have massages regularly, stop after the second month as deep massage of the pressure points can cause problems. Instead, light massage around the feet, legs, neck and shoulders and lower back can be extremely beneficial and you deserve it!

Late pregnancy massage oil
50ml grapeseed oil
4 drops essential oil of lavender
3 drops essential oil of Roman chamomile
3 drops essential oil of mandarin
50ml bottle

Mix ingredients together in the bottle and shake well. Use as a massage oil for backache after thirty weeks of pregnancy. This oil will keep for up to a month. ꙮ

Labour
Most women find giving birth daunting and it can be one of the hardest and most painful experiences in life but you can also make it one of the most wonderful. Women have different perceptions of what will happen so it is important to be well informed. Talk to your midwife or gynaecologist and ask questions – you want to be prepared!

I was lucky to be born in a room full of flowers that my grandmother had collected that morning. She was my mother's midwife and in that part of France it was the tradition to fill the room with fragrance so a baby's first breaths were of sweet-smelling air. My mother was also able to concentrate on the flowers and their fragrance, and breathe deeply.

Breathing

Obstetric practices vary from one place to another and you may want to ask about or rehearse some breathing exercises before labour. To help, put one drop of essential oil of petit grain, lemon or orange and one of neroli on a tissue and inhale when you do your breathing exercises. ❧

Room fragrance

Two weeks before you are due to give birth, fill your home with the fragrances of rose, neroli and mandarin – add a drop of each to a bowl of boiling water and breathe the vapours. The oils will help to ease breathing, totally relax and de-stress and act as a natural tranquillizer. Your baby will become familiar with the smell so you can bring the scent to the delivery room. Place a bowl by your bedside during labour to calm and relax. Get someone to replace the bowl after an hour, as the aromas will evaporate. ❧

Music

A favourite piece of music could be a relaxing accompaniment to the birth. Bring something with you that you listen to often and as the baby has heard it in the womb so he will be familiar with the sound. ❧

Labour massage oil

During labour, get your partner or midwife to rub a little of this oil on your lower back. It contains:

Neroli – good for the nervous system and helps you cope with mental exhaustion.
Petit grain – calming and brings clarity to a tired mind.
Mandarin – good for anxiety, a natural tranquillizer.

50ml grapeseed oil
2 capsules borage oil
1 capsule wheatgerm oil
1 capsule evening primrose oil
1 drop essential oil of neroli
5 drops essential oil of petit grain
4 drops essential oil of mandarin
50ml bottle

Mix ingredients together in the bottle and shake well. Rub gently over lower back, feet and hands. ❧

Bathing after labour

After your baby is born it is important to keep your genital area clean to prevent infection. A good way of doing this is to use coarse sea salt in your bath (but don't have it too hot!): fill a large jar with the salt adding five drops essential oil of tea tree, five drops essential oil of chamomile and two drops essential oil of rose. Put the lid on and shake well. Pour two tablespoons of this under running water and relax for at least seven to ten minutes. ❧

Oils to avoid during pregnancy

Sue Mousley from the George Eliot Hospital in Nuneaton, one of the UK's top midwives, has shared with me how she uses essential oils in her work in this chapter, and provided her recipe for the late pregnancy massage oil. The following list gives her guidelines for oils to avoid during pregnancy or to use only during labour. The reasons why are detailed in the list.

Carrot – regulates menstruation.
Clary sage – facilitates labour and is thought to quicken it, so best to leave for labour only. Mixes well with frankincense in a bath (six drops clary sage, four drops frankincense in 50ml natural, fragrance-free bubble bath).
Cypress and melissa – both regulate menstruation so best to avoid in pregnancy.
Geranium – large doses or frequent use can alter clotting mechanisms due to its anticoagulant effects, also a hormone balancer.
Jasmine – strong uterine tonic, again great for labour and as a pain reliever, helps deliver placenta if a little stubborn. Use as a compress to fundal area.
Lavender – only use after sixteen weeks of pregnancy with caution as it regulates menstruation and is a toner of the uterus.
Peppermint – thought to have oestrogen-like properties and may stimulate labour so I always avoid it in pregnancy. However, it is good to use in labour when many mothers suffer a lot of nausea.
Rose – strong uterine tonic, great though to facilitate labour and as a pain reliever.
Rosemary – raises blood pressure so avoid completely during pregnancy and labour.

Arms and elbows

Arms

Like everything else, the skin on the arms starts to sag as we get older. We may also notice cellulite, with its characteristic dimples, and the only real answer to the problem is exercise, although massage and the application of essential oils as described below will all help. Walking and running will improve the circulation in the arms, as will swimming (especially backstroke), which will tone and firm. Stretching exercises are good too and a gentle upward massage will also help lymphatic drainage.

Splashing cold water on the arms after a bath or shower will activate the circulation and a firming vinegar lotion is also useful. With continuous attention and daily applications of essential oils, you will see an improvement.

Massage oil for upper arms

Massage this oil into the triceps muscle in an upward movement. Regular use will help firm and tone the upper arm (but don't forget to exercise too!).

45ml (3 tablespoons) jojoba oil
10ml (1 dessert spoon) rose masqueta oil
1 capsule wheatgerm oil
1 capsule evening primrose oil
3 drops essential oil of either rose or jasmine
5 drops essential oil of lavender
4 drops essential oil of either bois de rose or lemon
100ml bottle

Mix together in the bottle. After a bath or shower, use the oil to massage the triceps muscle from the elbow upwards. This oil will keep for up to two months. ❧

Armpits

The strong odour sometimes associated with armpits is due partly to the fact that the body's elimination process takes time, which means the sweat is trapped under the armpits – hence the smell. There are also three different glands in the armpit area that are responsible for producing strong odours.

The first is the eccrine gland – a small sweat gland that regulates heat in your body. There are approximately 3000 million of these little glands around the body and, the hotter the weather, the more they secrete. The apocrine glands are slightly larger and found around the armpits, genital area and the nipples. These are responsible for body odours and secrete sweat in small spurts. (More sweat is produced when we are under physical exertion or stress.) When sweat is mixed with dead skin cells the odour gets stronger, and humid conditions (under clothing) provide the perfect environment for bacteria to multiply. If perspiration isn't washed away or neutralized the smell can become really unpleasant. Thirdly, the sebaceous glands produce a substance called sebum that contains fatty acids, natural waxes, protein and cholesterol. Hormones control the glands and if we are over-anxious, stressed or emotional they will secrete more.

These three glands control our body odour (this is also affected by pheromones, which can fluctuate during the female menstrual cycle) and if we allow these smells to linger we are deemed unclean. Sweat is very personal; it can be sweet and acrid or acidic and the way a person smells is often partly due to their health, diet, age, environment or time of the month. So much money is spent on deodorants as we are told from an early age that perspiring is bad. But we are spraying and rolling ourselves with chemicals that are bad for our health. Some suppress the natural secretions, some cause rashes and spots, and some have even been associated with breast cancer. After a while our bodies build up immunity to these chemicals thus rendering them less efficient anyway.

The good news is that essential oils really help eliminate these odours as they help slow down heavy sweating naturally, will not endanger your health and make you smell lovely too!

Natural gel deodorant

Clary sage will help slow down secretions and it is deodorizing too. You could supplement clary sage with angelica or rose oil.

2 tablespoons pectin powder
15ml (1 tablespoon) aloe vera juice
1 capsule wheatgerm oil
1 capsule evening primrose oil
8 drops essential oil of clary sage
2 drops essential oil of basil
2 drops essential oil of lavender
1 drop essential oil of peppermint

Make up the pectin as instructed on packet. Mix ingredients well and place into a small jar (make sure the lid is screwed on well). Leave for three days before use. Apply gel after a bath or shower, massaging a little under each armpit. This preparation makes enough for two to three weeks' supply. Keep in a cool place. ❧

Natural deodorizing spray

You can alternate between clary sage, angelica and rose oil. This handy bottle is to keep in your handbag.

50ml boiled water, cooled down
5ml (1 teaspoon) aloe vera juice
1 capsule wheatgerm oil
4 drops essential oil of clary sage
3 drops essential oil of lavender
3 drops essential oil of ylang-ylang
2 drops essential oil of vetiver
Spray bottle

Pour the ingredients into the bottle and shake well. Leave for a couple of days before using for the first time.

Shake well before use. This will keep for up to two months.

After-shaving lotion

Most women wax or shave their armpits regularly but if you suffer from extra-sensitive skin, soreness may develop soon afterwards. Geranium, tea tree, palmarosa, clary sage and myrrh are all good bactericide, antiseptic and deodorizing essential oils that will calm irritated skin.

200ml boiled water, cooled down
8 drops essential oil of geranium, tea tree, palmarosa, clary sage or myrrh

Add your chosen oil to the water and mix well. Rub the lotion on the armpit gently using a cotton wool pad. Repeat a few times and don't apply deodorant for a while. ❧

Elbows

Rough and dry elbows can be a real age giveaway so regular moisturizing is a must.

Cocoa butter moisturizer

Cocoa butter is a marvellous skin softener.

10g cocoa butter
5ml (1 teaspoon) avocado oil
1 capsule wheatgerm oil
1 capsule evening primrose oil
5 drops essential oil of palmarosa
50ml jar

Warm the cocoa butter, avocado, wheatgerm and evening primrose oils together over a bain-marie. When melted, remove from the heat and stir in the essential oil. Pour into a jar. Apply to the elbows every night before bed. Massage it in and leave on for ten minutes. Take off the surplus with a tissue. This will keep for up to two months. ❧

Elbow treatment

Gently scrub the elbows every day with a pumice stone or loofah. Follow with an application of this cream:

50ml pot fragrance-free (organic if possible) moisturizer
2 drops essential oil of bois de rose
2 drops essential oil of palmarosa
1 drop essential oil of lemon

Stir the oils into the moisturizer before gently massaging it into your elbows. ❧

Lemon bleach for elbows

Stand each elbow in half a lemon for a few moments. This is great for both lightening and softening the skin on the elbows. ❧

Protecting oil for elbows

If you enjoy lifting weights or doing push-ups it is important to warm your elbow joints up first.

5ml (1 teaspoon) grapeseed oil
8 drops essential oil of rosemary
5 drops essential oil of black pepper

Mix together and pour into a small bottle. Rub vigorously into elbow joints before exercise to warm them up. ❧

Hands and nails

Hands

Our hands can sometimes show our age more than our face. They are often the first thing people notice about us and, however fresh and young your face looks, if your hands are not cared for they'll give your age away. So often I see women with glowing, moisturized skin on their face and yet they have hands that seem to belong to a different person!

Our hands are on show all year round and need treating with as much care as our face, as they are in use constantly. They are incredibly precious to us, being the way we experience the world through touch, yet often we barely spare a second's thought to caring for them. They are exposed to pollutants, such as dirt, grease, strong hand creams, chemicals and washing-up liquid. They carry heavy loads and often come into contact with wind and rain. After time, sometimes during the menopause, ageing spots appear. The skin on the backs of our hands becomes thinner, looser and more wrinkled as collagen and elasticity are lost.

In the last ten years the market has been flooded with hand-care products but these tend to be loaded with chemicals. However, essential oils can really help. They are restorative and will keep your hands young looking too. Good essential oils to use on the hands are geranium, patchouli, rosemary, lime, lemon, lemongrass, carrot, sandalwood, tea tree and rose.

Basic rich hand cream recipe

This is a good rich, basic hand cream to share with all the family. It is really easy to make but it will require your full attention the first time you make it – it is definitely worth the attempt! This recipe requires ten drops of two different essential oils. I used tea tree and rosemary here, but you can alternate between the ones listed above.

15g organic beeswax
15g cocoa butter
30g (2 tablespoons) almond oil
2 capsules wheatgerm oil
4 capsules evening primrose oil
5 drops essential oil of rosemary
5 drops essential oil of tea tree
2 x 50ml jars

Use a bain-marie (see page 12) to slowly melt the beeswax and cocoa butter. Remove from the heat and add the almond oil and contents of both the wheatgerm and evening primrose oil capsules. (You can add more almond oil here if you want the cream to be more liquid.) When the mixture starts changing colour take off the heat, stir in the essential oils, and pour into two jars to set (one for home and one for your handbag). The hand cream will keep in the fridge for up to six weeks. ❧

Ageing spots

Ageing spots can appear from exposure to too much sun. Often called 'liver spots', they also appear with age. Try this massage oil:

15ml (1 tablespoon) almond oil
15ml (1 tablespoon) argan oil
1 capsule wheatgerm oil
2 capsules evening primrose oil
10 drops essential oil of lavender
2 drops essential oil of rose
50ml bottle

Mix together and shake well. Every evening, massage the oil into the hands until fully absorbed. This will keep for up to two months. ❧

Palmarosa rejuvenating hand mask

1 egg yolk
1 tablespoon white clay powder
1 capsule wheatgerm oil
6 drops essential oil of palmarosa
2 drops essential oil of cedarwood

Mix well with a spatula and apply on the top of hands with a make-up brush. Leave on for five minutes. Remove the mask by gently washing your hands in warm water. For extra-soft hands you can apply the following oil afterwards:

2ml (1/3 teaspoon) argan oil
1 capsule borage oil
1 capsule wheatgerm oil

10ml (1 dessert spoon) almond oil
10 drops essential oil of palmarosa
2 drops essential oil of mint
50ml bottle

Mix together and shake well. Massage a little of the oil into the hands, applying firm pressure with your fingertips. Use once a week. ❧

Moisturizing coffee grounds

This is a wonderful, quick hand reviver. After your morning coffee, retain the grounds. Transfer to a small bowl and add two drops essential oil of benzoin and one drop essential oil of rosemary. Stir well. Rub on hands for a few moments before washing off with warm water. ❧

Hand treatment for sore, rough hands

This is a great rich cream for sore hands (it is especially good for gardeners).

5g organic beeswax
5g cocoa butter
10ml (1 dessert spoon) castor oil
10ml (1 dessert spoon) linseed (flax) oil
30ml (2 tablespoons) jojoba oil
50ml orange flower water or rosewater
1 drop essential oil of either neroli or rose
4 drops essential oil of benzoin
4 drops essential oil of tea tree
200g pot

Melt the beeswax, cocoa butter, castor, flax and jojoba oils in a bain-

marie. Remove from the heat and stir in the orange flower water or rosewater and the essential oils. Pour into a small pot and massage into the hands when needed. This makes approx four to six weeks' supply. Store in a cool place. ❧

Warts

Warts are unsightly lumps often caused by viral infections. They are contagious and extremely difficult to get rid of. In my opinion, the best treatment for warts is an application of neat essential oil of either tea tree or ravensare. Apply your chosen essential oil to the wart once a day with a cotton bud. This is very effective but it may take a while so be patient.

Basil is full of wart-busting constituents and is also a useful remedy.

10ml (1 dessert spoon) almond oil
2 capsules wheatgerm oil
3 drops essential oil of basil
50ml bottle

Mix together and shake well. Apply to warts twice a day with a cotton bud. (If you're feeling adventurous you could apply a fresh basil leaf to your wart and cover with a plaster!) ❧

Nails

Many people in the medical and health-care professions regard the nails as a window to someone's overall health and lifestyle. A careful examination can reveal white spots, lack of colour, soft texture, vertical and horizontal lines, which can all

reveal a 'medical history'. So there is more to nails than the occasional application of hand cream and varnish, and acrylic extensions.

Nails are a hard surface made from the protein keratin with traces of phosphorus (you can smell it when you file them), calcium and traces of some metals. A good diet is extremely beneficial for nail health, especially important are vitamins A and E and protein. The good thing is that natural ingredients and essential oils will help to restore, rejuvenate and keep your nails looking good. Some of the best essential oils to use are rosemary, grapefruit, ravensare, galbanum, frankincense, marjoram, myrrh and patchouli.

Nail instruments can be a haven for bacteria so make sure you don't share yours with others. Before use, apply a drop of either tea tree, marjoram or ravensare to the scissors etc. using cotton wool. A small basket is the perfect place to store orange sticks, cotton buds, gentle nail files and wooden emery boards, nail scissors and a soft stone.

Short nails

I always prefer to keep my nails short, as they are easy to look after and keep nasty bacteria at bay. Cut them at least every five to six weeks to encourage their growth. This is best when the nails are slightly soft – after a bath or shower is preferable and don't forget to disinfect your scissors first! Keeping them all one length will give the appearance of healthy hands – don't forget that nails are an extension of your hands; they work in tandem to look good.

Brittle nails

Strong detergents and household products can be the cause of brittle nails that break easily. Always wear rubber gloves to do the washing-up and be sure to protect your nails when gardening. The resinous essential oils of frankincense, galbanum and myrrh work well here, so pick the one you prefer.

10ml (1 dessert spoon) linseed oil
1 capsule wheatgerm oil
2 drops essential oil of frankincense, galbanum or myrrh
50ml bottle

Mix together and shake well. Use the oil once a week, rubbing on individual nails to strengthen them. This will keep for up to two months. ❧

Cuticles

Cuticles are there to protect the nail and stop them getting infected by outside pollutants. They should not be cut! I have seen many patients who come to me with infected nails because of a bad manicure, cuticles cut to the quick and bleeding.

The best time to push cuticles is after a bath or shower when they have softened slightly. Dip your fingertips in a bowl of warm water containing a drop of essential oil of rosemary, patchouli, ravensare or grapefruit. Relax for a few moments before gently drying and using an orange stick to carefully push back your cuticles.

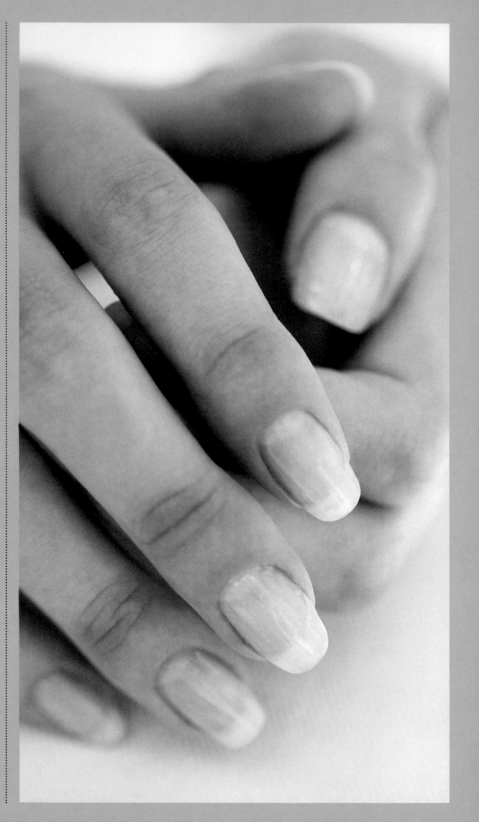

Buffing treatment

Healthy nails look their best buffed to a good shine. Invest in a good buffer; it will boost the circulation and add a nice, healthy pink colour to your nails. Daily buffing will also help strengthen the nails. This preparation is a good pre-buffing treatment. The inclusion of white clay helps draw out impurities and disinfect the nails.

1 tablespoon white clay powder
A little boiled water
5ml (1 teaspoon) almond oil
10 drops freshly squeezed lemon juice
2 drops essential oil of lemon

Mix the white clay powder with a little water in a bowl to obtain a paste. Stir in the almond oil, lemon juice and essential oil of lemon. Use an old toothbrush or a cotton bud to apply to each nail. Leave on for at least twenty minutes before rinsing off and buffing each nail. ❧

Nail shine and moisturizer

This is great for keeping in your bag for instant moisture and shine.

5ml (1 teaspoon) castor oil
1 capsule wheatgerm oil
1 drop essential oil of rosemary
50ml bottle

Mix together and shake well. Massage oil into nails last thing at night or after washing hands. This will keep for up to two months. ❧

Lemon cleanser

Keep your nails beautiful by dipping your fingers into a bowl of hot water with a few drops of lemon essential oil (or the juice of half a lemon). Lemon acts as a disinfectant, killing bacteria and it also helps bleach nails. Pat dry, and then clean under your nails with an orange stick. Again lemon is useful here, so wrap a little cotton wool around the tip of your stick and dip in the juice. Clean as before. ❧

Hand and nail treatment mask

This treatment is wonderfully restorative for both nails and hands. Apply this mask in the bath, as it is easy to wash off afterwards.

2 tablespoons Manuka honey
1 egg yolk
20ml (2 dessert spoons) avocado oil
1 capsule wheatgerm oil
1 drop essential oil of rosemary, patchouli, grapefruit or ravensare

Mix the ingredients together in a small bowl. Massage into each hand paying special attention to the nails. Leave on for fifteen to twenty minutes before rinsing off in the bath. Do once a week. ❧

Natural nail stain

This will last for a few weeks and act as a nail protector too. There are many henna colours available, so choose one that suits your skin tone. This looks especially good in the summer.

1 dessertspoon henna powder
A little boiled water
1 drop essential oil of patchouli

Add the henna powder to a small glass and make a paste with a little water. Stir in the essential oil of patchouli and apply to each nail using a cotton bud or a small brush. Let dry – if it's sunny you can dry your nails in the sunshine – this may take a while. Rinse off with warm water to reveal the pinky shade. Follow by buffing them to a shine. Apply a 'nail whitener' pencil underneath each nail tip. ❧

Lemon stain remover

Smoking discolours fingers and nails, but you can remove these unsightly stains with fresh lemon juice. This will act as a bleach and an anti-bacterial agent and disinfectant. Apply the juice with a small nail-brush, rubbing gently into your fingers and nails. ❧

Nail infections

The essential oils of tea tree, thyme, rosemary and ravensare are all good for nail infections. Keep tea tree in every time but you can alternate between rosemary, ravensare and thyme.

2 drops essential oil of tea tree
1 drop essential oil of rosemary
1 drop essential oil of ravensare
150ml boiled water

Stir the essential oils into the water. Leave to cool before dipping the nails into the solution for at least ten minutes. Dry gently. Use cotton wool to apply a drop of one of the oils neat to the infected nail(s). Use daily until infection has cleared up. ❧

BANISH CELLULITE & VARICOSE VEINS

Throughout fashion history the ideal female shape has changed. In the past people worshipped a more plump form, when breasts, hips and waists were in vogue.

Now we all want to be thin but I firmly believe that the most important aspect of beauty is health.

Women's body shapes change throughout their lifecycle – this is nature and natural and should be embraced rather than fought. But if we put on weight or lose it too quickly it will not only affect our health but also our skin, and can cause cellulite. At least nine in ten women, both those who are thin and those who are fat, are affected by it. It is much more noticeable as we get older and can make us very self-conscious.

Cellulite can be brought on by hormonal changes characterized by high levels of oestrogen. This encourages the body to retain fluid, causing the fat cells to bunch up and protrude through the dermis. The skin on the thighs, bottom, stomach or arms takes on a lumpy appearance, sometimes referred to as 'orange peel' or 'buttons on a mattress'.

Today most people in the medical profession agree that cellulite is different to normal fat and in some countries, such as France, it is looked upon as a medical condition. The French researcher Dr Belaiche thinks it could be caused by a dysfunction of the endocrine glands, resulting in more oestrogen (a hormone genetically programmed to store fat) being produced. The contraceptive pill could also be a contributor as it encourages the production of oestrogen. Smoking, alcohol, bad posture, not enough exercise, and a poor diet are other factors. Stress, both mental and physical, alters the way the body functions and as a consequence can prompt the storage of fat and affect the digestion. It is a constant battle, not helped by our twenty-first-century lifestyle!

The cellulite-busting products on the market today are in constant demand and as they are so readily available we are loath to change our bad habits. But we can try to improve these habits – take time to look at my solutions. I have studied and researched many plants and ingredients over the years, and have looked after many patients suffering with cellulite. In the mid-1980s, *Harpers & Queen* rated my cellulite oil very highly and I have formulated many products for High Street companies.

Cellulite-busting tips

Make sure you drink a lot of herbal tea during the day as many have natural diuretic properties. Good ones are: basil, peppermint, fennel, aniseed, sage, thyme, green tea, rosehip and gingko biloba. Also try rose tea, which will help regulate appetite. Fresh juices are also wonderful; try apple, celery, fennel or carrot. Increase your intake of vitamin C – rosehip, lemon and grapefruit are all good sources.

Eat plenty of organic green vegetables rich in iodine (seaweed, for example). This helps the thyroid gland in the production of hormones that regulate the metabolism. Interestingly, in Asian countries where seaweed (and soya) features heavily in the diet, cellulite occurs less frequently in women. Good green vegetables to add to your diet include: watercress, parsley, spinach and cabbage. It is also important to avoid sugary foods and foods high in salt. It seems that women least affected by cellulite have a healthy diet, rich in fish oils, and a lifestyle devoid of stimulants such as alcohol and coffee.

Wheatgerm oil (vitamin E) is wonderful – I add wheatgerm flakes to everything. Include pulses, whole grains and seeds in your diet too (fennel, coriander, caraway and fenugreek are all good). It is also important to cut down on dairy products. Eat plenty of food containing phyto-hormones (plant hormones), such as soya products (beans and tofu), yams, peas, sprouted seeds and grains. Think each time you put something in your mouth – do you really need it?

Take plenty of exercise regularly, as it helps to boost circulation. Stretching, toning, swimming, yoga, walking and dancing are all enjoyable and helpful. Exercise will help the body to burn the fat instead of storing it, reducing the fatty layer between the muscle and skin.

Take time to relax, since a relaxed body will be able to get rid of the toxins and waste accumulated more easily. Recharging your batteries is so important – take a nap in the afternoon, even ten minutes will be of benefit if you can manage it. Be aware of your breathing and take good deep breaths.

Skin brushing and exfoliating helps the lymphatic drainage, reducing the fat cells that cause cellulite. It will also improve the blood flow and limit free-radical damage. Invest in a loofah or a gentle bristle brush and massage and brush the skin in circular movements towards the heart. For more on this, see below.

How can essential oils help?

Essential oils contain phyto-hormones (plant hormones) and have natural diuretic properties and cleaning agents. They regulate capillary activity and restore vitality to the skin tissue, boosting a sluggish system. Day-by-day the traces of rejuvenating vitamins and minerals in essential oils can help us de-stress and relax, thus preserving our strength and youth.

Regular applications of essential oils will assist in the firming of those areas affected by cellulite. The following oils will give the best results:

Basil – this is wonderful for the nervous system and a natural diuretic.
Black pepper – this is warming and stimulates circulation.
Celery – like fennel, celery is a natural diuretic and can be useful for fluid retention. It can also assist with weight-loss.
Cinnamon – this is a strong antiseptic. It is a warming herb that stimulates circulation.
Clary sage – its plant hormones help rebalance the system and eliminate fat deposits.
Cypress – this is a wonderful detoxifier. Good for blood circulation and veins.
Fennel – this has long been regarded as a slimming herb and has natural diuretic properties. It helps fluid retention too.
Geranium – this is warming, stimulating and detoxifying.
Grapefruit – this is rich in rutin, which strengthens capillaries and traces of vitamin C; it is also detoxifying.
Juniper – this is excellent for fluid retention, a natural diuretic.
Lavender – this also benefits the nervous system and helps relax and de-stress.

Lemon – this is rejuvenating and detoxifying. Like grapefruit, lemon also contains rutin and traces of vitamin C.
Oregano – this is a warming herb with natural anti-bacterial properties.
Rose – this has a high vitamin C content and can help regulate the appetite. It is good for the heart, the blood circulation and can influence the female sexual organs. It also has a wonderful scent.
Rosemary – this rejuvenates and detoxifies.
Thyme – this assists with lymphatic drainage and stimulates circulation.

Cellulite treatment

This treatment consists of skin brushing, a scrub, followed by a detoxifying bath and finally a massage with an oil. If you don't have time to do everything, choose one or two parts of the treatment – every little bit helps!

Body brushing

Body brushing will undoubtedly help the fight against cellulite and will also improve the skin. Make sure the brush isn't too soft, since if it is it won't make a difference. Be gentle on the areas affected by varicose veins or broken capillaries, scars, cuts and skin problems. If your skin is extra-sensitive, brush it in the bath or under the shower where the friction won't be so hard. Always brush in the direction of the heart.

Start with the feet and brush up your legs, front and back. Brush the bottom and hips, focusing carefully on each area. Rub the stomach in both circular and long upward movements. Then do the back of the neck, shoulders and back of the arms.

Sea salt scrub

Before you get into the bath, massage the scrub in circular movements into the key areas. The bonus of coarse sea salt is that it is rich in iodine and a real detoxifier. This is enough for two to three baths.

500g coarse sea salt
10ml (1 dessert spoon) avocado oil
1 dessert spoon runny honey, Manuka if possible
2 drops essential oil of geranium
2 drops essential oil of either rosemary or cinnamon
2 drops essential oil of black pepper
Jar

Mix together and put into a medium-sized jar. Take a handful of the scrub and massage it into the affected areas – pay special attention to the backs of the thighs, hips and shoulders (you may have to get someone to help you!). Rub in circular movements, taking care around varicose veins and broken skin. Use the scrub twice a week. 🦶

Detoxifying bath essence

This essence is wonderful in the evening or after a heavy session at the gym, a long walk or a hard day at work. It really relaxes and detoxifies and contains a high concentration of essential oils – you can pick your favourites and alternate between them. **Note:** If you suffer from

varicose veins or broken capillaries don't have the bath too hot.

50ml grapeseed oil
1 capsule wheatgerm oil
1 capsule evening primrose oil
10 drops essential oil of fennel
10 drops essential oil of lavender
10 drops essential oil of either oregano or thyme
10 drops essential oil of eucalyptus, pine, niaouli or cajuput
10 drops essential oil of either cypress or juniper
100ml bottle

Mix together in the bottle and shake well. Pour a capful/tablespoonful under running bath water. Relax for at least ten to fifteen minutes. This essence will keep for up to six months. 🦶

Massage oil

This oil contains guarana. This acts as a lipolytic enhancer, meaning it activates the circulation and stimulates the blood flow. The oil will need to stay on the surface of the skin for a few minutes before you massage it in. **Note:** You will need to shake the oil well before every application, as the contents will separate.

10ml (1 dessert spoon) aloe vera juice
20ml (2 dessert spoons) almond oil
60ml grapeseed oil
10ml (1 dessert spoon) guarana tea or 2–3 dissolved capsules guarana
2 capsules wheatgerm oil
1 capsule borage oil
5 drops essential oil of either thyme or fennel

6 drops essential oil of rose
10 drops essential oil of lemon, grapefruit or orange
10 drops essential oil of either cypress or violet leaves
100ml bottle

Pour ingredients into the bottle and shake well. Massage into affected areas daily. This will keep for three to four weeks in a cool, dark place. 🦶

Leg massage oil

If your cellulite is only really at the top of the legs, try the following massage treatment.

50ml grapeseed oil
1 capsule borage oil
1 capsule wheatgerm oil
2 drops essential oil of cypress
2 drops essential oil of clary sage
2 drops essential oil of lemon
1 drop essential oil of orange
2 drops essential oil of rosemary
1 drop essential oil of violet leaves
50ml bottle

Mix ingredients together in the bottle and shake well. Make sure you are sitting comfortably on a towel on the floor, with one knee bent, and massage from the knee towards the hip using firm pressure (although never squeeze the skin too hard). Finish by using circular movements towards the hips on the top, insides and back of the thigh. Repeat on the other leg. Use the oil morning and night for a month then reduce to two or three times a week afterwards. This oil will keep for two to three months. 🦶

Varicose veins

Often cellulite is accompanied by bad circulation and the appearance of varicose veins in the legs. These are caused by interruptions of the blood flow. People who stand a lot are more susceptible to the condition, as are those who don't exercise or exercise too strenuously. It is also a genetic condition.

Bath essence

20ml (2 dessert spoons) grapeseed oil
2 capsules evening primrose oil
1 capsule wheatgerm oil
4 drops essential oil of cypress
2 drops essential oil of either parsley
   or violet leaves
4 drops essential oil of lavender
3 drops essential oil of wintergreen
1 drop essential oil of peppermint
1 drop essential oil of either pine or
   lemon
50ml bottle

Mix together in the bottle and shake well. Add one capful per bath but don't make the bath too hot! Follow with an application of the massage oil below. Use twice a week. This essence will keep for up to six months. ❧

Massage oil for varicose veins

45ml (3 tablespoons) grapeseed oil
20ml (2 dessert spoons) almond oil
1 capsule wheatgerm oil
1 capsule evening primrose oil
5 drops essential oil of either parsley
   or violet leaves
5 drops essential oil of cypress
4 drops essential oil of either
   lavender or lemon

4 drops essential oil of either pine or
   wintergreen
2 drops essential oil of peppermint
100ml bottle

Pour the ingredients into the bottle and shake well. Massage into legs once a day in an upward direction. Keep in a cool place. This will keep for four to six weeks. ❧

Green tea lotion for varicose veins and leg cramps

This is a really good massage oil for veins and cramps. Use after sport or a bath or shower.

200ml strong green tea
50ml aloe vera juice
1 capsule wheatgerm oil
1 capsule evening primrose oil
1 drop essential oil of peppermint
5 drops essential oil of lavender
5 drops essential oil of cypress
2 drops essential oil of parsley
4 drops essential oil of orange
½-litre bottle

Mix ingredients together in a bottle. Leave for two days. Shake well before use. Massage oil into legs in an upward direction two or three times a week. This preparation is enough for two weeks' supply. Keep in a cool place. ❧

Preventing varicose veins in pregnancy

(See also pages 116-119.) To avoid varicose veins in pregnancy, it is very important to rest as much as possible with your feet up, even if it is just for ten minutes. Place a flat cushion under your neck and another under your knees. Breathe deeply and fully to encourage the circulation – make sure the window is slightly open in the room where you relax so you get plenty of fresh air. You could even take advantage of this time to meditate and think positive thoughts about the future.

Vitamin-rich massage oil

The following oil is great for preventing varicose veins and will also help if you already have varicose veins or thread veins. All the ingredients are rich in vitamin C and rutin which will help to strengthen capillary walls. Geranium will encourage good circulation and the citrus oils will have a slightly astringent effect upon the whole venous system. The aroma is also very positive and uplifting. You should also make sure that you eat a diet rich in fruit and avoid hot baths or carrying heavy loads.

50ml soya oil
1 capsule wheatgerm oil
2 drops essential oil of geranium
2 drops essential oil of grapefruit
1 drop essential oil of lemon
1 drop essential oil of orange
50ml bottle

Mix ingredients together in the bottle and shake well. Stroke the oil very gently into the legs using upwards movements, from the feet to the thighs. Use daily. The oil should keep for two to three months. ❧

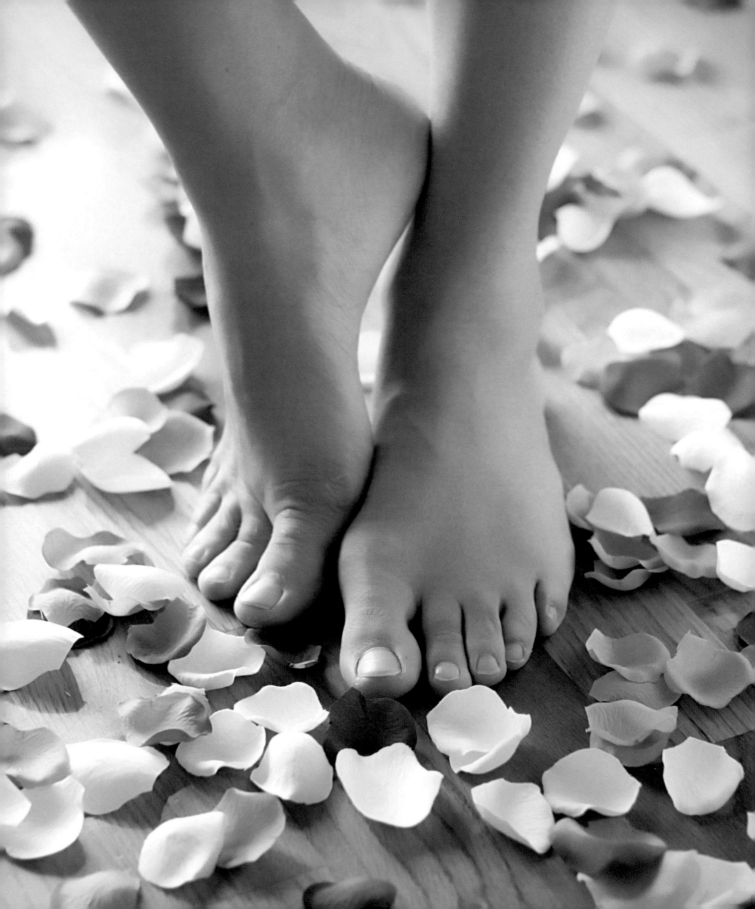

Feet

Unfortunately our feet are often neglected; other parts of our bodies take priority and feet are considered ugly by some people. But our feet are so important! They are constantly under pressure – carrying us everywhere; carrying our weight day by day. Our busy, active lives are only possible because of our feet and we only start to notice them when they swell up, smell and hurt. Only then do they get our attention. Some researchers believe that Man was originally meant to walk on all fours and that the foot and back problems we experience today are a consequence of walking on two feet!

A decade ago I spent time in Mexico with a group of friends. One night on the beach they decided to do some fire walking on a small fire they had started. Some of them were experts at walking on hot charcoal but I had had no experience, so at first I was wary. My friends persuaded me that it was a wonderful way to discharge negative energy and 'ground' the static accumulated in the body over the past year. After the drumming and chanting I felt I had to do it and presented myself to the 3m (10ft) length of charcoal. To this day I can't remember walking over the coals; I just disconnected for a few minutes. When I realized what I had done I

felt so great – light and on top of things. I talked with my friends afterwards and I was so excited to have overcome my fear. It is incredible how the heat travels through your body, all the way to the top of your head. Even to this day when I visualize that time the feeling of the lightness comes back.

Obviously fire walking is quite dangerous but walking barefoot on grass and sand are not and they are just as beneficial too. They are perfect for releasing built-up tension and great for toning every muscle and ligament. Invest in a good volcanic pumice stone to help smooth hard skin and treat yourself to a new pair of nail clippers. Almond oil is great softening oil for the feet. By pampering your feet on a regular basis you can eliminate toxins and improve the circulation.

Essential oils are a wonderful treat for the feet and they all have bactericidal properties. Some have cooling properties, such as peppermint, which helps neutralize odours; some help the circulation, such as clary sage and pine; others have wonderful fragrances, such as lavender and vetiver (which are also antiseptic); and some are both antiseptic and disinfecting, such as lemongrass. Thyme, black pepper and rosemary are also good because they have warming qualities.

Tired feet

Always try to elevate your feet at the end of a hard day. Lie with your back on the floor and prop them up on the sofa or chair, or lie on the sofa resting them on the arm. Keep this position for ten to fifteen minutes – it's great for draining away fatigue and increasing circulation.

Cypress footbath for tired feet

This footbath is wonderful after a long walk; it soothes sore feet after a day in high heels or too much dancing or sport. It is also good for sweaty feet.

12 drops essential oil of cypress
10 drops essential oil of lavender
5 drops essential oil of mint
1 tablespoon natural, fragrance-free
  liquid soap, shampoo or bath foam

Add the essential oil drops to the soap, mix and then add this solution to a bowl of hot water. Submerge your feet and relax for ten to fifteen minutes. ❧

Pampering foot treatment

Over 72,000 nerve endings finish at our feet! No wonder a foot massage makes us feel so relaxed and light, and our whole body will benefit from it. Begin with a relaxing footbath – fill a large bowl with warm water and add two drops essential oil of lavender and two drops essential oil of clary sage. Mix and submerge both feet for at least ten minutes. Dry both feet carefully, toe by toe; all humidity must be removed otherwise the feet will be susceptible to athlete's foot and other fungal infections. Finish with a foot massage using the oil below. I've used lemongrass and pine here but you can alternate between the others.

5ml (1 teaspoon) almond oil
1 capsule wheatgerm oil
1 drop essential oil of lemongrass
1 drop essential oil of pine

Mix together before massaging into both feet. Take your time and enjoy!

Lavender and sage massage oil

If you've been on your feet all day or perhaps had a long session at the gym a foot massage may be just what you need. The combined oils of lavender and sage have a soothing action and you will instantly feel relief from swelling and blisters. It works especially well after a bath or shower.

10ml (1 dessertspoon) grapeseed oil
1 capsule wheatgerm oil
18 drops essential oil of lavender
3 drops essential oil of sage

Mix together, then rub the oil vigorously into the feet for a few minutes (be gentle on blisters and swelling). Make sure you massage the soles and between the toes. Do this twice a week.

Hydrating oil for very dry feet

This oil is especially good after a footbath containing a couple of drops of clary sage, lemongrass or lavender and a cup of aloe vera juice.

30ml (2 tablespoons) aloe vera juice
5ml (1 teaspoon) castor oil
1 capsule wheatgerm oil
8 drops essential oil of clary sage
8 drops essential oil of lemongrass
2 drops essential oil of lavender

Mix together before massaging the oil into both feet. Do this twice a week until skin improves.

Sweet-smelling shoes

Put a few drops of your favourite essential oil onto some tissue paper, scrunch it into balls and push them into your shoes. Keep in overnight for sweet-smelling tootsies!

Athlete's foot

Athlete's foot is a contagious fungal infection and can be accompanied by itching between the toes, redness, a rash, split and flaky skin. It is the area between the toes that is most affected so always make sure you dry them properly – athlete's foot thrives in damp, humid places. Footwear should be aired regularly (particularly trainers), and walking barefoot whenever you can would be beneficial. The infection is quite a nuisance and precautions must be taken to protect other members of your household – be rigorous about using separate towels and, if it gets too bad, consult a podiatrist.

Oil for athlete's foot

10ml (1 dessert spoon) soya oil
1 capsule wheatgerm oil
8 drops essential oil of lemongrass or patchouli
5 drops essential oil of peppermint
50ml bottle

Mix ingredients together and pour into the bottle. Apply to the affected area every day. Make sure you massage the oil between the toes and around the toe-nails. These amounts make enough for one month.

Excessive sweating and athlete's foot

Clary sage, lemongrass and tea tree oils are very effective for this. Alternate between them. Add two drops of your chosen essential oil to a bowl of warm water. Submerge the feet for at least ten minutes. Then carefully dry the feet as before. Finish with an application of this oil:

5ml (1 teaspoon) soya oil
1 capsule wheatgerm oil
3 drops essential oil of either lemongrass or lavender

Mix ingredients together and massage the feet, toes, between the toes and the sole for a few minutes. Take the surplus off with a damp towel. Use three times a week.

Bunions

Bunions are painful and obtrusive inflammations of the joint between the toe and the foot. Common causes are ill-fitting shoes, so always wear the correct size and width for your feet. The following foot rub is helpful too.

Peppermint foot rub
5ml (1 teaspoon) grapeseed oil
2 drops essential oil of peppermint

Mix together and rub into the feet well. This is particularly good at the end of a long, hot day! ❧

Corns and hard skin
These are often caused by bad posture and inappropriate footwear. Use a pumice stone after a footbath to remove excess skin. Then follow with the following oil.

Softening oil for corns
5ml (1 teaspoon) avocado oil
5ml (1 teaspoon) castor oil
1 capsule wheatgerm oil
1 drop essential oil of lavender
1 drop essential oil of jasmine

Mix ingredients together and massage into both feet. Use every day for a week, then twice a week. ❧

Softening foot mask
If you have more time, you could try this remedy. Yarrow is a wonderful astringent and softener.

50ml of a strong yarrow infusion
1 tablespoon white or green clay
*   powder*
5ml (1 teaspoon) castor oil
1 capsule wheatgerm oil
1 drop essential oil of lavender
1 drop essential oil of jasmine

Prepare the yarrow infusion using a tablespoon of yarrow in 250ml boiling water. Let cool and strain. Mix the clay with the yarrow infusion to form a paste. Add the castor oil, the wheatgerm capsule and the essential oils. Apply to the top and bottom of each foot and leave for fifteen minutes. Rinse off, dry each foot carefully and apply the softening oil above. ❧

Foot scrub
Use this scrub once a week to prevent hard skin and corns forming.

1 handful coarse sea salt
5ml (1 teaspoon) sesame oil
2 drops essential oil of lavender

Mix together in a little bowl. Rub the feet vigorously with the scrub, massaging them for a few minutes. Then plunge into a footbath containing a few drops of one of the foot-friendly essential oils. ❧

Blisters
Blisters are painful swollen areas often caused by new shoes. If a blister bursts you will need to keep it clean and free of infection. Bathe it with cooled down boiled water containing a little sea salt and a drop of geranium, eucalyptus or tea tree essential oil.

You could also try this solution:

½ cup of a rosemary infusion
5 drops essential oil of rosemary,
*   cypress or lavender*

Prepare the rosemary infusion using two sprigs of fresh rosemary and 250ml boiling water. Let cool and strain. Mix in the essential oil. Use a cotton bud to apply the solution to blisters. Use two to three times a day and store in the fridge. ❧

Chilblains
Chilblains are often caused by bad circulation and can affect any part of the body exposed to cold, particularly the toes. Chilblains are red, swollen lumps and can itch terribly. Rub neat geranium oil into them for instant relief.

Cold feet
Add a few drops of either black pepper, rosemary or tea tree essential oil to a basin of hot water. Dip a flannel into it, wring out gently and apply the hot compress to the feet.

Swollen feet
Swollen feet will benefit from a cooling gel containing peppermint.

1 tablespoon pectin powder
100ml strong peppermint infusion
3 drops essential oil of peppermint

Follow instructions for the pectin to obtain a gel. Make the peppermint infusion using two tea bags or a handful of fresh mint in a large cup of boiling water. Leave to cool and strain. Stir into the pectin with the essential oil. Massage into the feet in upward movements towards the heart. Leave on for fifteen minutes before rinsing off. Use twice a day. ❧

ENJOYING EXERCISE TO THE FULL

Living in large cities and leading stressful lives, leads to us constantly being exposed to physical and emotional pressures.

This can lead to laziness and we can be tempted to turn to drink or drugs in order to relax. But we need to learn to enjoy simpler pleasures instead – walking or biking in the park for instance.

Physical exercise instantly relieves stress, anxiety and, in some cases, even fatigue. It will encourage efficient circulation of the blood and will ensure a good intake of oxygen – twenty-five to thirty minutes of exercise a day is all you need. Exercise is vital for our health as it strengthens the underlying muscles and promotes good breathing, and both these will go a long way to maintain a good posture. Another welcome benefit of exercise is that it will help to keep you feeling and looking young!

Swimming, cycling and dancing will all help tone the thighs, bottom and legs, while skipping and boxing are great for the heart. Walk regularly, in the countryside, near the sea or in a park – don't always rely on cars and public transport to get around. There are so many fun forms of exercise out there and you can even share them with a group of friends to encourage each other's efforts. It is really important to choose an exercise that is right for you, and that is one that you enjoy doing. There is nothing worse than doing an exercise that you don't enjoy – it must be pleasurable and fun! Don't be put off by the odd aches and pains – sometimes even laughing or walking can be hard. When you are unfit, your muscles are bound to feel tired. This will get better and wear off after a couple of days – ready for the next time! The benefits far outweigh the pain. Remember that exercise will keep you fit and active. It will also perk you up, de-stress you and improve any sleeping problems.

Exercise and breathing

Did you know that each person takes approximately 23,000 breaths a day? Old Chinese texts said that 'your age corresponds to how many breaths you have had in your life'. So breathing is the dynamic to stay alive and exercise activates breathing, thus helping your health. In order to stay young and healthy, it is important to learn how to breathe deeply and fully.

If you find it difficult to breathe during or after exercise, essential oils can help you. Eucalyptus, pine, niaouli, cajuput and tea tree are all particularly good for the lungs as they clear the respiratory system and purify the air around you, helping to kill unwanted germs.

The following essential oils are also great for assisting with exercise and promoting energy. They will encourage deep breathing, blood flow and circulation – great companions to have around! Rub a little of your chosen oil on your chest and torso before exercise (if you have sensitive skin put a drop of your chosen essential oil in a teaspoon of grapeseed oil before applying to skin). Alternatively, if exercising at home, put a few drops in a bowl of boiling water and place near you when exercising.

Cajuput – helps the lungs and respiratory system, aids breathing.
Eucalyptus – good for respiratory system, lungs, aids detox.
Mandarin – good for nerves and mental stress.
Marjoram – energizing, with anti-bacterial and antiseptic properties.
Neroli – helps anxiety and nervousness, calming.
Niaouli – helps the lungs and respiratory system.
Petit grain – aids mental stress.
Pine – good for respiratory system, lungs, aids detox.
Rosemary – energizing, with anti-bacterial and antiseptic properties.
Tea tree – good for respiratory system.

Exercise and meditation

Consider learning to visualize and meditate to help your exercise routine. Also select from yoga, t'ai chi or Pilates – all of which are good for strengthening the muscles. Choose an exercise that feels right for you and incorporate some meditating essential oils into your practice (frankincense, sandalwood, rose or neroli). Meditation, with the right essential oil, makes you start visualizing and it is such a great way to relax.

Before exercise meditation

Add a few drops essential oil of frankincense, sandalwood, rose or neroli to a bowl of boiling water. Place near to you when meditating, inhaling deeply. You could also make a massage oil – add a few drops of essential oil to a carrier oil and massage into torso, solar plexus and under nose. ❧

After exercise shower

Add a few drops of a relaxing essential oil to the shower tray and shower as normal, breathing in the fumes. Alternatively rub a few drops of essential oil into your torso and under your nose, then shower as usual, breathing deeply. ❧

Baths to take after exercise

Foam or salt bath for aches and pains

This bath is wonderful for those post-exercise aches and pains. If you prefer a bubble bath, use shampoo; alternatively you can use sea salt.

Natural, fragrance-free shampoo or coarse sea salt
4 drops essential oil of rosemary
3 drops essential oil of cypress
2 drops essential oil of pine
2 drops essential oil of lavender
Eggcup

Fill an eggcup with shampoo or coarse sea salt. Stir in the essential oils and pour under running bath water. ❧

Epsom salts bath for aches and pains

Epsom salts are renowned for easing aches and pains. Relax in this bath half-an-hour before bed.

75g Epsom salts
3 drops essential oil of petit grain
6 drops essential oil of lavender
2 drops essential oil of melissa
2 drops essential oil of neroli

Mix ingredients together and add to the running bath water. Make sure you inhale the fumes, breathing in and out deeply. Concentrate on your breathing and relax for ten minutes. Afterwards, wrap yourself in a warm dressing gown and relax on your bed until you fall asleep. ❧

Cedarwood bath oil for aching muscles

The bubble bath acts as an emulsifier, enabling the essential oils to disperse more easily. The oils in this bath can work against digestion so it's best not to eat until a few hours afterwards.

5–10ml (1–2 teaspoons) of natural, fragrance-free bubble bath
10 drops essential oil of cedarwood
5 drops essential oil of pine
5 drops essential oil of juniper

Mix the oils with the bubble bath, add to a warm bath and relax. ❧

Massage rubs

Massage rub before exercise

Lemon is great for sport as it induces sweating and has an antiseptic and deodorizing action.

50ml grapeseed oil
2 capsules wheatgerm oil
15 drops essential oil of lemon
50ml bottle

Mix ingredients in the bottle and shake well. Massage into legs, arms, torso and solar plexus (in a clockwise direction). This oil should keep for two to three months. ❧

Therapeutic rub for aches and pains

Massage into affected areas after an exercise session. It also helps toning and relaxation.

30ml (2 tablespoons) soya oil
30ml (2 tablespoons) grapeseed oil
1 capsule wheatgerm oil
3 drops essential oil of rosemary
2 drops essential oil of pine
2 drops essential oil of tea tree
4 drops essential oil of ylang-ylang
3 drops essential oil of geranium
50ml bottle

Mix together ingredients in the bottle before massaging into muscles. Concentrate on the nape of the neck, shoulders and upper arms, spine and lower part of the back, feet and legs (always massage in the direction of the heart). After your massage, dip a towel in hot water, wring and place it on your back – bliss! This oil should keep for two to three months. ❧

Massage rub after exercise
Lemon goes well with rosemary and marjoram and, used together, they stimulate and tone up the body.

50ml grapeseed oil
1 capsule wheatgerm oil
7 drops essential oil of rosemary or marjoram
8 drops essential oil of lemon
50ml bottle

Mix ingredients in the bottle and shake well. Massage into legs, arms, torso and solar plexus (in a clockwise direction). This oil will keep for two to three months. ❧

For sports injuries
The following oils should all keep for two to three months. (It can be difficult to find good quality camphor of borneol oil so check carefully with your supplier.)

Oil for joint stiffness
Chamomile combined with camphor of borneol is great for easing joint stiffness.

10ml (1 dessert spoon) soya oil
1 capsule wheatgerm oil
12 drops essential oil of Roman chamomile
8 drops essential oil of camphor of borneol
Eggcup

Mix ingredients together in an eggcup. Rub the oil gently on the affected parts for a few minutes. ❧

Juniper massage oil
This will encourage circulation and strengthen the capillaries, veins and muscles.

30ml (2 tablespoons) soya oil
2 capsules wheatgerm oil
10 drops essential oil of juniper
5 drops essential oil of lemon
6 drops essential oil of cypress
50ml bottle

Mix together in the bottle and massage into the affected areas. Use two to three times a week. ❧

Cypress massage oil to stimulate circulation
10ml (1 dessert spoon) almond oil
1 capsule wheatgerm
3 drops essential oil of cypress
2 drops essential oil of sage
1 drops essential oil of mint
50ml bottle

Mix together in the bottle. Massage into the soles/tops of your feet every day. This is also great for swollen ankles. ❧

Massage oil for painful joints
10ml (1 dessert spoon) almond oil
1 capsule wheatgerm oil
3 drops essential oil of cedarwood
3 drops essential oil of marjoram
2 drops essential oil of peppermint
50ml bottle

Mix well in the bottle and massage into affected area twice a day until pain goes. ❧

Massage oil for tennis elbow
The very common and extremely painful condition known as tennis elbow can occur when one is too enthusiastic about tennis, weight training or other exercise. Long periods at a computer can also cause pain in the elbow, as can diseases such as rheumatoid arthritis. The tendons on the outer part of the elbow become inflamed and tender, causing a lot of discomfort and pain. They take time to heal, as there are fewer blood vessels in that area, so massage is important. Combined with essential oils, this will improve circulation and aid healing. You will need to generate heat in the elbow area so make sure you rub in the massage oil vigorously.

45ml (3 tablespoons) grapeseed oil
10ml (1 dessert spoon) castor oil
1 capsule wheatgerm oil
5 drops essential oil of rosemary
5 drops essential oil of juniper
2 drops essential oil of black pepper
5 drops essential oil of nutmeg
100ml bottle

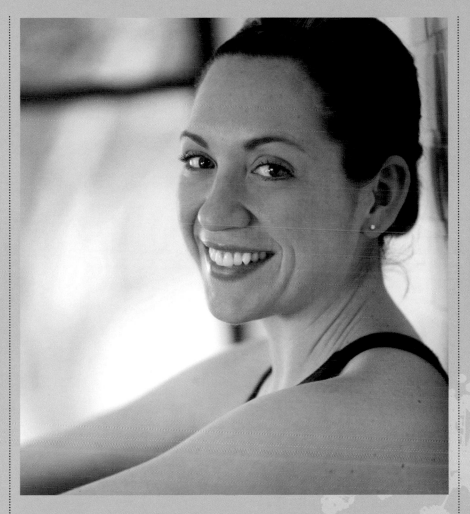

Mix together in the bottle and rub the oil vigorously on the affected parts for a few minutes. Use as needed. ⚘

Massage oil for aches and pains

20ml (2 dessert spoons) soya oil
2 capsules wheatgerm oil
10 drops essential oil of aspic
2 drops essential oil of thyme
50ml bottle

Rub this oil on affected areas, repeating after one hour if the pain is bad. Continue treatment when needed. This is particularly good after a warm bath. ⚘

Juniper footbath

Essential oil of juniper is very useful in the treatment of aching joints or sports injuries (twisted ankles etc). It is particularly good in footbaths – add six drops of essential oil of juniper and two drops essential oil of cypress to a large bowl of hot water. Submerge feet and relax for five to seven minutes. This footbath will help to reduce swelling and aching. ⚘

Cramp

If you are often plagued by cramp, try walking barefoot on a cold floor (cold tiles are particularly good). This will help cramp in the calf muscles.

Avoid tea and coffee, drinking instead infusions of thyme. Add B vitamins to your diet, and take two teaspoons of either wheatgerm or flax oil per day.

Drink pure cranberry, black grape or blackcurrant juice regularly.

Mix the ingredients together and pour into the bottle. Apply the oil with a vigorous massage twice a day, one hour before a bath or shower, half-an-hour before bed. This will keep for up to three weeks in a cool place. ⚘

Protecting oil for elbows

If you enjoy lifting weights or doing push-ups it is important to warm your elbow joints up first.

5ml (1 teaspoon) grapeseed oil
8 drops essential oil of rosemary
5 drops essential oil of black pepper
50ml bottle

Mix together in a small bottle. Rub vigorously into elbow joints before exercise to warm them up. ⚘

Chamomile and rosemary oil for aches and pains

30ml (2 tablespoons) soya oil
2 capsules wheatgerm oil
8 drops essential oil of Roman chamomile
4 drops essential oil of rosemary
50ml bottle

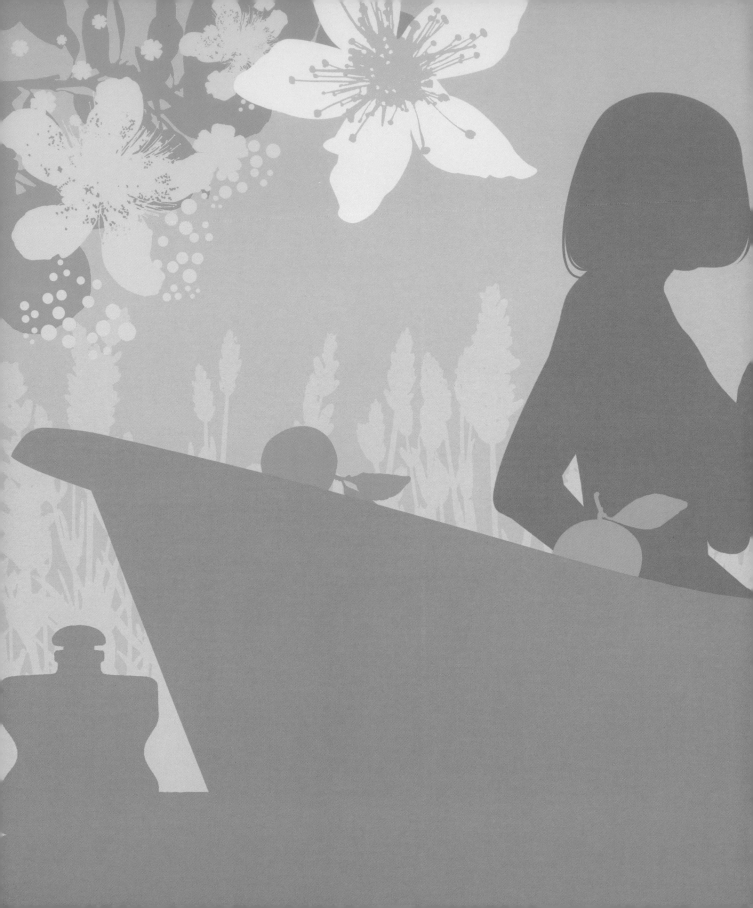

part three
PAMPERING

Bathing

A bath with added essential oils is a special therapeutic and rejuvenating treatment. The revitalizing aromas will create a wonderful experience for your senses and help you recharge your batteries, de-stress, relax, aid sleep and detox; some can even help slimming and rejuvenate. Depending on what essential oil you use, you reap its particular benefits.

Bath treatments are so easy to make at home and are quick too – only ten minutes' preparation. In total you will need about half-an-hour for a whole treatment and that will include fifteen minutes' relaxation time in the bath. Any more time and your skin will dehydrate. This is also the case if your bath is too hot – it may be tempting in the winter months but a really hot bath can increase your chances of getting broken veins and capillaries. It will also put a strain on your heart and circulatory system so you could end up feeling nauseous and faint.

Aromatic bath tips

Always run the hot water for a while before adding the essential oil, shut all the doors and windows so you keep the fumes within. Use your hands to disperse the essential oils in the water, four to six drops per bath is enough. Have a quick shower first to wash; you don't want to add unwanted soapy products to your nice bath!

Never have a bath after a heavy meal as this will disrupt your digestive pattern and could make you feel dizzy. You will not benefit at all. I don't advise using foaming bubble baths as they often contain chemicals and unwanted preservatives, and can cause allergic reactions. If you can't go without bubbles make sure you choose a natural brand.

Remember to relax for at least ten minutes after your therapeutic bath. Lie on your bed or sofa in your dressing gown and cover your eyes with cotton wool pads dipped in flower water. Follow with an application of your chosen body oil.

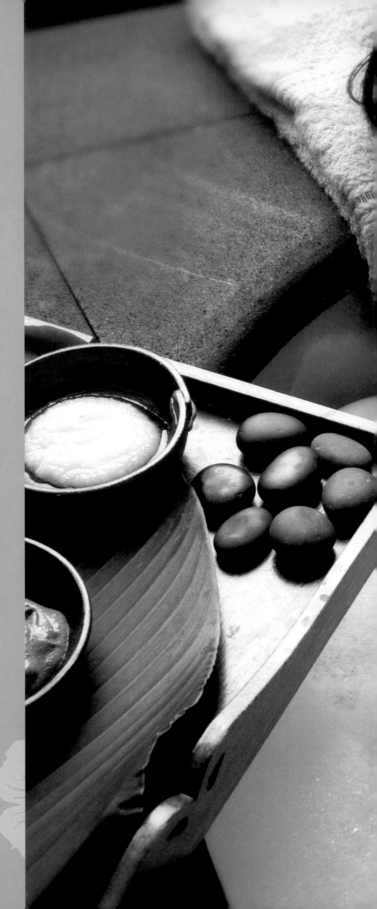

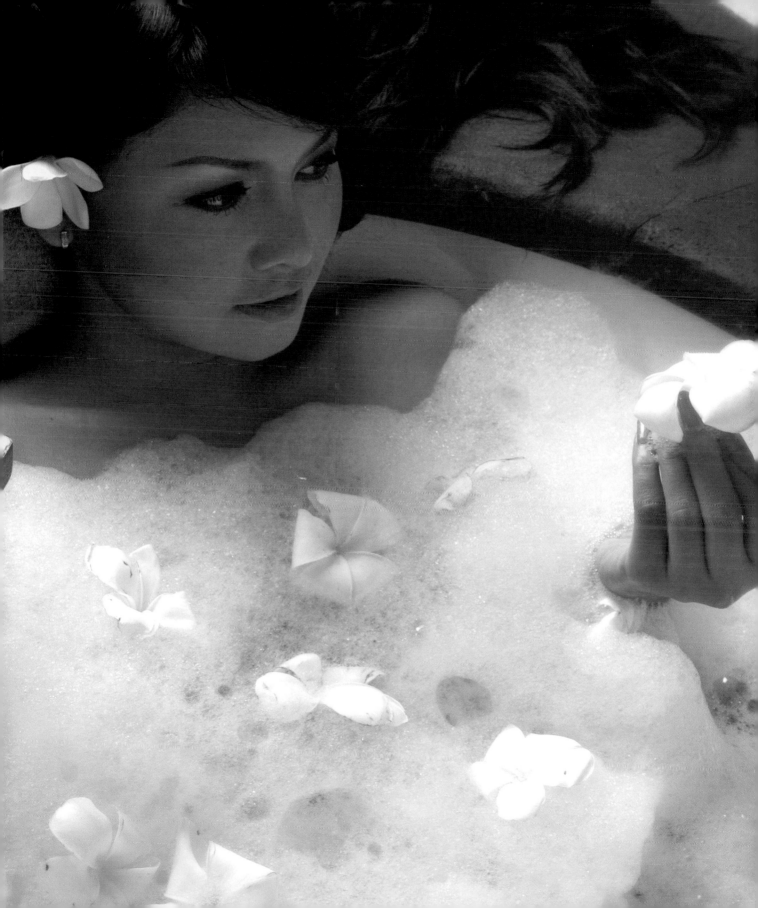

Royal milk bath

Immerse yourself in a milk bath just like Cleopatra did. You can use whole milk or dried milk powder – both are wonderful for the skin.

*600ml (1 pint) organic whole milk or
  equivalent amount of milk powder
3 drops essential oil of rose
2 drops essential oil of orange
1 drop essential oil of either patchouli
  or sandalwood*

Stir the essential oils into the milk and pour under the running water, mixing in well. Relax for fifteen minutes. ❧

Detox bath

This is great after a late night out or if you have had too much alcohol.

*2 large handfuls coarse sea salt
4 drops essential oil of lemon
1 drop essential oil of fennel
1 drop essential oil of juniper*

Mix ingredients together and add to running water. Relax for fifteen minutes. Use a loofah to rub your thighs, feet, legs, stomach, back of the neck and shoulders. (Alternatively you can exfoliate before the bath.) ❧

Exotic bath

*1 cinnamon stick
5 cloves
½ vanilla pod
600ml (1 pint) boiling water
3 drops essential oil of ylang-ylang
2 drops essential oil of bergamot
1 drop essential oil of jasmine*

Add the spices only to the boiling water. Take off the heat and cover. Leave overnight so you end up with a strong infusion. Add to your bath water with the essential oils. Relax for fifteen minutes. ❧

Milk and honey bath

This will make your skin feel really soft.

*600ml (1 pint) whole milk
2 tablespoons Manuka honey
1 drop essential oil of chamomile
1 drop essential oil of carrot
4 drops essential oil of bois de rose*

Stir the honey and the essential oils into the milk. Pour under running water and relax. For extra smooth skin you can rub extra honey on your elbows, feet, knees and breasts before getting into the bath. ❧

Seaweed bath

Seaweed is packed with minerals and is also a natural pick-me-up. It can be obtained from any good health food shop.

*½ packet dried seaweed
5 drops essential oil of cypress
2 drops essential oil of lavender*

Wash the seaweed then soak it in a little water to soften. When softened, remove the seaweed and add to your running bath with the essential oils. Relax for fifteen minutes. If you are not too keen on sharing your bath with seaweed you can always make a juice. Add the dried seaweed to

600ml (1 pint) of water and bring to the boil. Simmer for approximately ten minutes, reducing liquid by half. Let cool, and then add this 'juice' to your bath with the essential oils. ❧

Spirulina bath for aches and pains

Powdered spirulina can be obtained from any good health food shop. It is rich in minerals and great for aches and pains.

*4 tablespoons spirulina powder (or
  more if your bath is big!)
3 drops essential oil of rosemary
2 drops essential oil of juniper
1 drop essential oil of cedarwood
1 drop essential oil of lemon*

In a bowl, mix the spirulina powder into a paste with a little water. Stir in the essential oils and pour under the running bath water. (**Note**: This bath is very green and may stain towels so use a dark one!) ❧

Epsom salts bath

This bath is great for relieving tiredness after exercise. It also helps aches and pains.

*200g Epsom salts
2 drops essential oil of geranium
2 drops essential oil of lavender
2 drops essential oil of ylang-ylang
2 drops essential oil of juniper*

Add the essential oils to the Epsom salts. Pour under running water, stirring to disperse. Relax for up to fifteen minutes. ❧

Honeymoon bath

Definitely for special occasions only! Buy three or four bottles of champagne and add to your bath when it's half full. Keep half a bottle for yourself (or for you and your partner) to drink! Add five drops essential oil of ylang-ylang, two drops essential oil of nutmeg. Mix well and add a little more hot water. Champagne is full of minerals and is great for the skin. ❧

Rejuvenating oil for dry skin

If you suffer from dry skin it is good to apply some body oil before you get in the bath. Massage it in and the warm water will then help its absorption, as well as protecting and treating the skin. Good essential oils to use are carrot, palmarosa, lavender, petit grain, rose, bois de rose and frankincense. Choose two oils for each batch, three drops of each. I have used lavender and petit grain here.

45ml (3 tablespoons) almond oil
1 capsule primrose oil
1 capsule wheatgerm oil
1 capsule borage oil
3 drops essential oil of lavender
3 drops essential oil of petit grain
50ml bottle

Mix ingredients together. Massage into your skin and then get in the bath. Relax for fifteen minutes. This should be enough for four to five applications and will keep for up to two months. A quick alternative is to use almond oil on its own. Massage into your skin as before then get in the bath. This will also work well. ❧

Body toning tonic spray

These sprays are fantastic, so toning and energizing. Select an essential oil for your purpose; maybe you want to relax, de-stress or calm yourself down. You can make up a couple of different sprays, one for energizing and one to relax – remember to put labels on your bottles! They are good for oily skins as they don't leave a residue on the skin surface. My grandmother used them regularly after therapeutic baths and she had a few to choose from on her dressing table.

5 drops essential oil of lavender
2 drops essential oil of peppermint
2 drops essential oil of lemon
3 drops essential oil of mandarin
3 drops essential oil of grapefruit
15ml (1 tablespoon) vodka (strong proof)
50ml cider or white wine vinegar
250ml mineral water
100ml jar
Large spray bottle

Mix your selected essential oils together in a small bowl and add the vodka. Stir well. Leave for twenty minutes to settle before pouring in the vinegar and stir again. Leave to settle for another twenty minutes then strain the liquid through a coffee filter into a jar. Put the lid on and leave to rest for ten days in a dark place. Transfer the scented liquid to the spray bottle and pour on the mineral water. Shake well. Spray over your body after a bath. This will keep for up to two months. ❧

Reviving cold bath

If you're feeling brave you may want to try a reviving cold bath. These are excellent; make sure you choose essential oils that energize, for example: two drops essential oil of rosemary, two drops essential oil of lemon and two drops essential oil of juniper. This combination is especially good in the summer months as it is very refreshing. ❧

Showers

If you don't have a bath or are in a hurry you may want to try an aromatic shower instead. They will make you feel refreshed and invigorated – a great way to start the day!

Before turning on the water, put four drops of an essential oil in the shower tray. Rosemary, juniper, lemon, grapefruit, pine, eucalyptus and peppermint all work well but it depends on how you want to feel. You can also rub a drop of your chosen oil on your torso, around your sinus area, nape of the neck and lower back. Turn on the shower and inhale the fumes, making sure you dry yourself vigorously with a towel afterwards. Follow with the body toning tonic spray, described above. ❧

BEAT FATIGUE; REGAIN VITALITY

Fatigue can result from too much stress, exercise, over-exertion, drinking too much or after viral infections.

Environmental pollution can also be a factor. We know that we can boost our energy with the right food and exercise, and having an active and attentive mind will also go a long way to energize and help us maintain our youthful looks.

Relaxation and recreation from work will also help us to regain energy, as will the use of aromatherapy and essential oils. Adding essentail oils to your bath or shower is a great way to regain your balance and prepare yourself mentally and physically for the day ahead. And a dynamic massage can equally refresh mind and body.

Revitalizers

Revitalizing body oil

Ginger, rosemary, peppermint and juniper are all wonderful oils to help revitalize the body and mind.

30ml (2 tablespoons) almond oil
30ml (2 tablespoons) soya oil
1 capsule wheatgerm oil
5 drops essential oil of rosemary
2 drops essential oil of peppermint
  or ginger or juniper
100ml bottle

Mix all the ingredients together in the bottle before massaging the whole body. Ideally use every morning after your bath or shower when you need a boost. The oil will keep for two to three months. ❧

Revitalizing bath essence

10ml (1 dessert spoon) grapeseed oil
20 drops essential oil of rosemary
10 drops essential oil of either juniper
  or ginger
5 drops essential oil of peppermint
50ml bottle

Mix together in the bottle and use five or six drops in the bath. Relax for up to fifteen minutes. For a shower, rub a little of the oil on your torso first.

After your daily bath or shower you can massage a little more of the oil on the nape of the neck, shoulders, feet and lower part of the back. Lie down for ten minutes and relax, with a pillow under your knees. Use for up to a week in times of need. The oil will keep for two to three months. ❧

Bath oil

This oil is mixed with an emulsifier to help it disperse in water (otherwise it just floats on the top!).

10 drops essential oil of chamomile
5 drops essential oil of ylang-ylang
Emulsifier such as a little bubble bath
  or some liquid soap (both natural,
  fragrance-free); if you're feeling
  adventurous – an egg!

Add to your morning bath to energize you for the day. Follow by a cold shower to stimulate circulation. ❧

Palmarosa bath or shower oil

15 drops essential oil of palmarosa
5 drops essential oil of lavender
A little natural, fragrance-free
  bubble bath

Add to your bath and relax for fifteen minutes. This oil will help calm you down and relax you. If you prefer a shower, make an oil to use in the shower from 15ml (one tablespoon) almond oil, five drops essential oil of palmarosa and three drops essential oil of lavender. Rub on torso, neck and solar plexus, massaging in for a few minutes. Follow with a shower, breathing in the vapours. ❧

Anti-fatigue rub

For an instant boost, try this quick rub.

10ml (1 dessert spoon) soya oil
2 drops essential oil of rosemary
2 drops essential oil of eucalyptus
1 capsule wheatgerm oil

Mix ingredients together and apply under your nose. around the sinus area or on top of your chest. Inhale deeply. ❧

Tonics and pick-me-ups

I swear by these good old-fashioned tonics for alleviating stress and fatigue and for aiding convalescence. They are particularly helpful for periods when you may be run down.

Tonic

In an old wine bottle, mix one-quarter strong chamomile tea (cooled down) with three-quarters sherry. Add one cinnamon stick and one-quarter teaspoon of grated nutmeg. Leave the bottle in a dark place for two weeks. When ready have a small glass a day. This is recommended for periods of stress and fatigue. It will keep for three to four weeks in a cool place. ❧

Orange tonic

1 litre white rum or vodka

1 kg orange peel, dried in a cool oven for a couple of hours

4 tablespoons brown sugar

2 cinnamon sticks

3 cardamom pods

Add ingredients to the bottle of alcohol. Leave in a dark place for fifteen days. Drink daily – add a little to a glass of white wine, water or tea. It is also wonderful added to cake mixtures and puddings. This tonic is good after a cold or flu. It will keep for up to a year. ❧

Orange pick-me-up

Peel the skin of an organic orange and place in a saucepan containing 600ml (1 pint) of boiling water. Add half a handful of orange leaves (available from health food shops, herbalists or ethnic supermarkets) and bring back to the boil. Remove from the heat and infuse for ten minutes. Cool and drink, adding honey to taste. This is wonderful for improving the memory and aiding concentration as well as being useful when you are feeling run down or convalescing. ❧

Rosemary wine

To relieve mental tiredness and distress, make a rosemary wine, by chopping 50g fresh organic rosemary and add it to three-quarters of a bottle of white wine (Sauvignon Blanc or Chardonnay). Shake well and leave in a dark cupboard for four days. Drink a small glass a day. This will last up to two weeks stored in the fridge. You can also pour into an ice-cube tray and freeze. ❧

Marjoram wine

This wine will help exhaustion and stimulate circulation. Add two-and-a-half tablespoons of fresh or dried marjoram to a bottle of good sweet red wine (madeira or Dubonnet for example) or sherry. Leave for a week in a dark place. Drink a small glass when feeling exhausted. This will last up to a month if well corked. ❧

Inhalation

If you're feeling depressed or have low self-esteem put a few drops of geranium essential oil into a bowl of boiling water. Sit close by and relax for a few moments with your eyes closed, breathing in deeply and holding and exhaling for three seconds each. The deep breathing combined with the essential oil will act as a tonic to the nervous system. ❧

Instant aid

In moments of need, these two quick tips will work wonders!

Study aid

Students will find essential oil of basil or lemon useful when studying. To aid concentration, add a few drops to a bowl of hot water and breathe in the fumes. ❧

Calming aroma for exhaustion

Add three drops of essential oil of sandalwood, basil or peppermint to a bowl of hot water. Mix and place next to you, relax. You can also add three drops to a spray bottle of boiled, cooled water, shaking well, and spray the air around you for an instant relaxing smell! ❧

The art of massage

Massage is one of the most ancient forms of healing and it is still our natural instinct to rub ourselves when hurt. Receiving a good massage is such an enjoyable experience and can be extremely beneficial and more therapeutic if essential oils are incorporated. Massage can help you to relax, de-stress, improve the circulation and assist with lymphatic drainage, encouraging the release of toxins. It will also promote a feeling of well-being – you will feel younger, revived, energized and full of vigour.

The therapeutic aspect of massage, however, does depend on the strength, length of time given, technique and the movements used. The rubbing action (if done correctly) will activate the nerve endings and warm up the skin – perfect for the penetration of the essential oils.

Massage naturally involves the sense of touch and if you practise regularly your fingers will soon be able to determine the areas that are tense. The small, remedial movements should come to you naturally – the hands should be firm and the fingers supple. Massage can be done to the face, back, chest, top of the hands, arms, legs and soles of the feet, and it is not too difficult. Try it on your family, friends and loved ones; you can even do it on yourself! Be cautious if someone is ill or pregnant, however, and consult a trained masseuse for guidance.

Some dos and don'ts of massage

Keep your nails short and always wash your hands first before starting a massage.

Never have a massage straight after exercise. You will be sweating as the body is eliminating toxins, so to ask it to reverse this and start taking in oils will be too much! Always have a shower before a massage as this will remove dirt and sweat, allowing better penetration of the essential oils.

If you find a good masseuse you can always ask them to use your own personal massage oil from one of the recipes in this book.

Massage techniques

Effleurage

This is the most used massage technique and it requires long, soothing strokes so you are slowly warming up the skin ready for the absorption of the essential oils. Place your hand flat and push it up on the skin. If you do this fast for a short time (ten minutes is enough) you will energize the recipient (or yourself). Use energizing massage oils containing rosemary, marjoram or eucalyptus.

If you want to calm someone down and relax them use slow movements, stroking the skin gently. Their muscles will start to relax and tension will be released, promoting a feeling of relaxation. Use calming massage oils made with neroli, rose, mandarin, Roman chamomile or petit grain.

Petrissage

These kneading movements are good for the fleshier parts of the body such as the tops of the legs and the hips. For this massage the thumbs are used more, slowly holding and releasing the skin. Petrissage improves the lymphatic flow.

Back massage

The healing properties of essential oils can provide some relief to bad backache or chronic pain. The oils will penetrate deep tissue and encourage the muscles to relax. The spine is one of the most important parts of the body and is an extension of the central nervous system from the

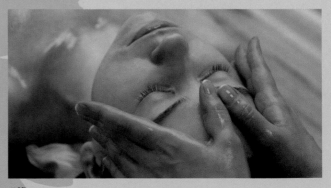

Effleurage

brain, so it will need to be given special attention. Use your hands to press down on either side of the spine, stroking upwards in parallel – excellent for stress and fatigue.

Head massage

This is so beneficial and very good to help relaxation. Use one of the relaxing oils for this (see above) – dip your fingers in a mixture of grapeseed and your chosen essential oil (see massage oil below). Only use a tiny amount otherwise you'll need to wash your hair! Use your fingertips to massage the back of the head first, slowly moving towards the top. Press the head gently with your fingertips. This is so good after a hard day's work.

Neck massage

This massage will benefit those who regularly carry heavy loads or office workers who lean over computers. Start at the base of the neck, using small, gentle, circular movements. Work either side of the vertebrae, then up the side of the neck to the base of the scalp. Continue for a couple of minutes, repeating the movements if there is particular tightness and stiffness in an area.

Shoulder massage

Use the two techniques of effleurage and petrissage as described above. Massage the muscles gently with the palms of the hands (the thumbs can also be used). Go with your movements from the base of the neck to shoulder and back again. Massage the shoulders with a good petrissage motion – your aim is to relieve the tension and knots in those areas.

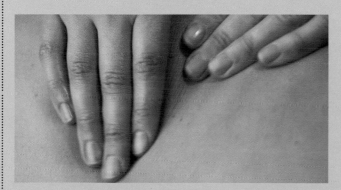

Petrissage

Arm massage

Use effleurage to massage up the arms to the top then under the armpits. Use petrissage around any muscular areas, but gently – if cellulite is present it can be painful!

Leg massage

If you are massaging yourself, do one leg at a time. First rest your leg on a small stool, starting with the feet and massaging upwards towards the heart. Use effleurage movements with gentle petrissage for any muscular or veiny areas or those with cellulite.

If you are giving a massage to someone else – place a small pillow under their knee. Start from the base of the leg, massaging upwards towards the knee, then from the knee to the top of the leg, front and back. Remove the pillow when you are doing the back of leg, placing a small towel for support under the front of the foot. This is especially helpful when there is tension in the back.

Foot massage

First warm up the area by placing a hot compress on each foot. The massage should start under the arch of the foot, continuing to the heel – this promotes good blood flow and encourages circulation. Massage around the ankles a few times, stroking the top of the foot. Then the toes – press each of them then release the pressure. Always support the foot with the other hand.

Simple massage oil

Choose an essential oil to relax or one to energize, depending on how you feel. Half an eggcup should be enough for a whole body massage and you can add wheatgerm oil if your skin is very dry.

½ eggcup soya or grapeseed oil
1–2 drops essential oil (depending on how large or small the person)
1 capsule wheatgerm oil (optional)

Mix ingredients together in the eggcup adding the wheatgerm if required. Massage the oil into the whole body for between fifteen and thirty minutes. ❧

ENHANCE YOUR SEX LIFE

We tend to take our sense of smell for granted, depending on more apparently significant senses such as sight and hearing. We feel sympathy for those who cannot see or hear but do we ever stop to consider how equally devastating it can be to lose our sense of smell?

Sex and the sense of smell

To me, sex and the sense of smell are very much interlinked. Humans, like animals, produce odoriferous substances called pheromones from the apocrine glands that lie just beneath the skin, which are there to identify and attract the opposite sex (and in animals also to mark their territory). The apocrine glands are found around the breast, genital, anal and underarm areas and also on the soles of the feet. The pheromones bring about all kinds of physical changes, they mix with sweat and send messages around us, radiating in the air until others pick them up. Yet, most of the time we are totally oblivious to their influence!

Animals use their pheromones as a form of communication to send messages to each other, marking territory, telling others of their destination and sexual status. For animals, the purpose of pheromones lies in sexual attraction and ensures the survival of the species. In ancient times, primitive man used his sense of smell to a much greater extent than we do nowadays. We see smell as a rather primitive function and most people rarely refer to it.

Yet research has shown that both men and women are responsive to each other's pheromones (men produce a musky scent whereas women produce a much sweeter smell), and that a woman's sensitivity to a man's scent soars or plummets with the fluctuation of her sex hormones.

The study of the sense of smell is called osmology, from the Greek *osma* or 'smell'. To me, a sharp, educated sense of smell is an incredibly valuable and pleasurable possession. It amplifies enjoyment and sensuality, extending desire and giving another dimension to love. This is, of course, well known to perfumers who are constantly asked to create perfumes that make people more attractive to others and even they depend on extracts from animal glands (or synthetic substitutes) to create the perfect scent.

Our sense of smell is engrained within us, our pleasures and our sexual desires. The nerves stimulated by different smells send messages to the brain and can unlock long-lost memories – for instance the scent of an aftershave can evoke the memory of a one-time lover. The memories all come back at once and still every detail can be conjured up after so many years. Essential oils can therefore add to this pleasure, enhancing desire, emotion and love. With oils we can create an impulse in the thought process, which can help the level of desire – and with the right aroma, the desire suddenly becomes achievable. Although we are not exactly talking about a love potion, a certain aroma can help the coordination of thought processes between mind and body.

The following oils are all good used in inhalations (add one drop to a bowl of boiling water), in the bath (use five drops under running water) or in massage oils.

Good stimulating essential oils for women are:
Rose, clary sage, sandalwood, jasmine, rose, bois de rose and tuberose.

Good stimulating essential oils for men are:
Cedarwood, ylang-ylang, nutmeg, neroli, sandalwood and black pepper.

Stimulating desire

A period of stress or emotional upset can affect the level of a person's desire and increase the body's requirements for certain nutrients and stimulating smells. All seafood is reputed to increase desire and sexuality, while peppercorns are considered to be an aphrodisiac by many ethnic communities. Ginger has a good reputation too – use it in cooking or drink in a tisane. Women who have lost interest in sex are advised to take angelica roots (in a tisane, see page 11), while many Russians swear by the aphrodisiac properties of caviar, oysters and vodka. **Note:** Alcohol drunk in large quantities can depress the central nervous system and lessen sexual desire.

On the fragrance front, Cleopatra tried to seduce Antony by lying on a floor covered in a layer of rose petals more than an inch thick. Imagine how wonderful and welcoming the aroma would have been! You, too, could try bringing flowers into a bedroom – tuberose, jasmine and hyacinths are all very effective.

Ginseng aphrodisiac

Ginseng root has aphrodisiac properties and is frequently used in Chinese medicine: cooking with it is a must if you want to increase your sexual appetite as it greatly enhances the libido. Alternatively, put a few ginseng root slices in a bottle of vodka or whisky and leave to infuse in a dark place for two weeks. Drink a small glass when the mood takes you. ❧

A love potion

Ylang-ylang is excellent for those who need a little aphrodisiac. A massage with this oil is especially good after a bath or shower but if you haven't got time to bathe first, prepare the body with a loofah to warm your skin to aid better penetration of the oils.

30ml (2 tablespoons) almond oil
5ml (1 teaspoon) argan oil
2 capsules evening primrose oil
3 drops wheatgerm oil
12 drops essential oil of ylang-ylang
50ml bottle

Mix the ingredients in a bottle and shake well. Then, for a few minutes, massage the oil into the lower part of the back, nape of the neck, ankles and feet. Do this every evening for a few weeks.

In addition to this, try adding five drops of ylang-ylang to a warm bath. Make sure the oil has dispersed well and jump in. The oil will start activating circulation within five minutes. This oil will keep for two to three months. ❧

Aphrodisiac bath oil

2 drops essential oil of black pepper
5 drops essential oil of ylang-ylang
2 drops essential oil of jasmine
1 drop essential oil of cedarwood
A little, natural fragrance-free shampoo
Eggcup

In an eggcup, mix the essential oils and the shampoo together. Pour

under running water and relax for up to ten minutes (your partner can jump in too!). Drink a glass of champagne in the bath to make you relax (but a whole bottle may make you fall asleep!). ❧

Aphrodisiac massage treatment

Follow your bath with a massage using this body oil. Touch is another very important sense and is heightened when two people are in love. Massage will help to unlock the emotions and make the experience more memorable.

45ml (3 tablespoons) almond oil
2 capsules wheatgerm oil
5ml (1 teaspoon) rose masqueta oil
2 drops essential oil of black pepper
2 drops essential oil of peppermint
4 drops essential oil of nutmeg
5 drops essential oil of ylang-ylang
2 drops essential oil of jasmine
50ml bottle

Mix ingredients together in the bottle and shake well. Use a little oil to massage your feet (you could massage each other's feet at the same time), back of the neck, temples and solar plexus. Massage the lower part of the back in circular movements for a few minutes. Relax. This oil will keep for two to three months. ❧

Creating a healthy environment

Essential oils at work

A recent survey in a national newspaper highlighted the unhygienic state of our workstations – apparently women have the dirtiest desks! If you are working hard and tend to eat lunch at your desk, crumbs and splashes can get into your keyboard and across the surface of your desk. In the confined space of your work area it is extremely important for your well-being to make sure it is as pleasant as possible.

Essential oils can not only help to stimulate your mind, but can also unwind and de-stress you, and give you the sense that you are pampering yourself at work. The importance of smells cannot be over-estimated and sweet-smelling things can really make a difference in our lives. Often the simplest ideas are the best – a small bowl of pot pourri near your desk, for example, can bring health benefits, boost your mental energy after hours in front of a computer screen and also help mask other unpleasant odours in the atmosphere.

Pot pourri

Place pine cones, freshly dried roses and freshly dried rosemary in a little bowl on your desk. To revive the aromas from time to time add one drop essential oil of rose, one drop essential oil of thyme and one drop essential oil of rosemary. This will make the pot pourri therapeutic as well as stimulating and reviving you. (It is always important to bring the outside world in when you are confined to a desk all day.) ❧

Natural cleaner

100ml boiled water, cooled down
5 drops essential oil of either geranium or bergamot
10 drops essential oil of rosemary
2 drops essential oil of either pine or basil
100ml spray bottle

Add the ingredients to the spray bottle and shake well.

Use to spray the surface of your desk every day and polish with a soft cloth. You can also use it to freshen up the air in a boardroom after a meeting and it works well as a hand cleanser too – spray your hands before and after lunch to get rid of germs. It will keep for up to two weeks. ❧

Pick-me-up

This pick-me-up is great after a few hours spent in front of a computer screen. Put a drop of essential oil of rosemary or geranium in your hands and rub together vigorously. Place your hands over your nose and breathe in the fumes for a few moments. ❧

Fragrant paper strips

Cut out strips of coloured paper and put a drop of a different essential oil on each (put the drop at the end of the paper). Try one drop essential oil of geranium, one drop essential oil of rosemary, one drop essential oil of pine and one drop essential oil of basil. Stand the paper strips up in a mug and place on your desk – inhale! ❧

Inhalation for sore eyes

If you've been staring at the computer for too long, or indeed if you have been driving for a while – this is a good remedy. If you wear contact lenses, remove them first.

Place a couple of drops of essential oil of chamomile in a bowl of hot water. Cover your head with a towel and inhale, opening your eyes intermittently so the vapours have a chance to go in. Finish by splashing your eyes with cold water. ❧

Essential oils at home

Recent research in Australia has linked the increase in childhood allergies with chemicals in household cleaning products. Some evidence links certain components in cleaning products with acceleration in the growth of breast cancer cells. I am certainly not surprised by these reports as I have seen more and more patients with allergies and respiratory problems in recent years.

The good news is that there are many natural alternatives to those strong, chemically based products. They are environmentally friendly, healthy and can even be more effective for cleaning! Essential oils have excellent anti-bacterial qualities and their natural alcohols mean they also have the perfect scent for use in the kitchen – and their aromas won't clash with the smell of food. Additionally, these natural scents will create an atmosphere of well-being and indulgence in your home and act as an instant pick-me-up too!

Kitchen cleaner

20ml (2 dessert spoons) cider vinegar
4 drops essential oil of lavender
4 drops essential oil of thyme
4 drops essential oil of lemon
4 drops essential oil of either eucalyptus or pine
4 drops essential oil of cedarwood (optional)

Fill a bucket half-way with boiling water then add the cider vinegar and the essential oils. Stir. This is wonderful to clean the kitchen surfaces, floor, wooden tables etc. You could also add it to a spray bottle to make surface-cleaning easier. Everything will shine! ❧

Kitchen cleaner

I always use essential oil of lemon to clean and disinfect my kitchen surfaces. Use undiluted or add a few drops to a bowl of boiling water. No need to rinse; it will evaporate naturally. The fresh citrus smell is wonderfully uplifting. ❧

Bathroom cleaner

This is great for clean, fragrant bathroom sinks and baths although you can also use it to clean smaller personal items such as nail scissors, tweezers and hairbrushes. Good essential oils to use are lemongrass, lemon, marjoram, thyme, tea tree or geranium. Choose two and mix 10ml (1 dessert spoon) of each (for example 10ml geranium and 10ml lemongrass) into a bottle and shake well.

Fill a bucket half-way with boiling water, mixing in a little fragrance-free washing-up liquid to make a foam. Stir in twenty drops of your essential oil mix and use to clean the sink, bath and toilet areas. Leave a few moments before rinsing off. Put a few drops of your chosen essential oils (neat) onto a towel or cloth and use to dry the surfaces and taps etc. ❧

Room perfume

Add five drops of essential oil of ylang-ylang to a bowl of boiling water and, within a few minutes, every room will smell amazing. If it's a special occasion you may want to float some eucalyptus, sage or basil leaves on the top for a really uplifting experience. ❧

Air freshener

Add a handful of eucalyptus leaves, five drops essential oil of pine and five drops essential oil of eucalyptus to an old saucepan of boiling water. Simmer slowly on the stove so the steam dissipates through the house. This helps to remove odours such as cigarette smoke from curtains and soft furnishings. Fresh eucalyptus leaves also help remove bad smells and are a passive smoker's friend! ❧

A scented wardrobe

Rolled-up balls of blotting or tissue paper impregnated with ten drops of essential oil of cedarwood make clothes and shoes smell heavenly (it also keeps insects and moths at bay) – just place the paper balls at the bottom of your cupboard or in your shoes for sweet-smelling toes! You can also try cypress, lavender or bois de rose. ❧

Sweet-smelling bed linen

My grandmother used to do this regularly – add forty drops essential oil of lavender and five drops essential oil of cedarwood to a tin of natural furniture wax. Mix well with a spatula then leave open in your linen cupboard for sweet-smelling linen. (This also acts as an insect repellent.)

Or, put ten drops of your favourite relaxing essential oil (lavender, petit grain, orange or ylang-ylang) onto a towel and add to your tumble dryer with your bed linen. You can look forward to a wonderful night's sleep. ❧

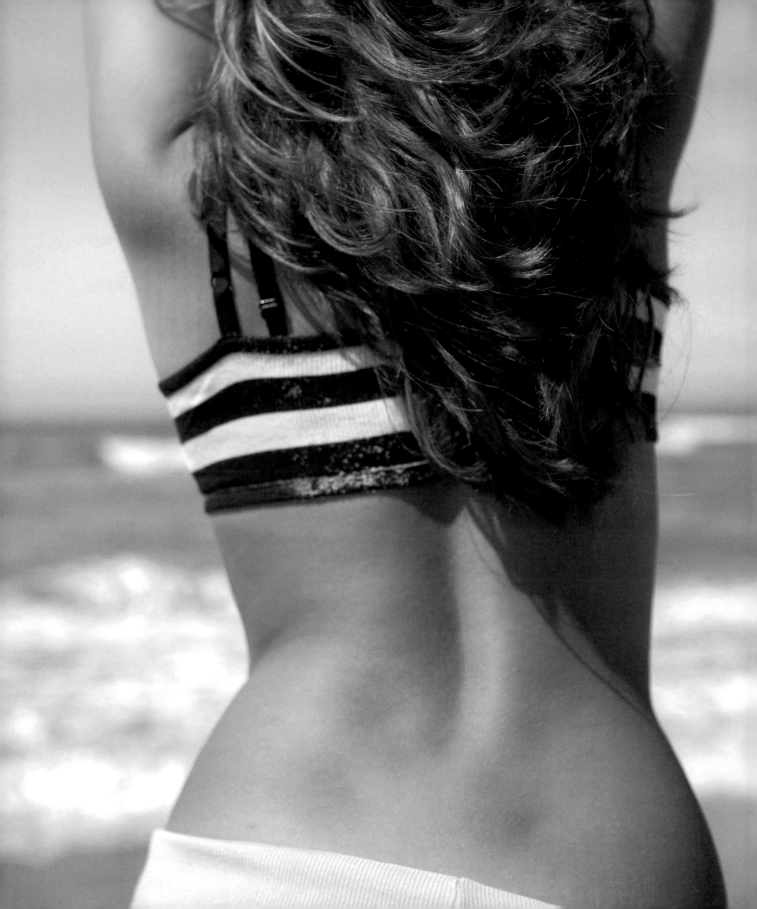

Pamper and protect yourself on holiday

Holiday sunshine

We are warned constantly in the media about the dangers of the sun, and dermatologists regularly talk about the serious effects it can have on our skin. Exposure to the sun is one of the biggest causes of skin cancer but still people sunbathe without protection. In the summer many of us in the northern hemisphere take to our beaches and parks, and we just lie there prostrate. On the other side of the world, Australians and New Zealanders, on the other hand, have been taught from an early age to 'slip, slap, slop'. Those in the southern hemisphere are more aware of the damage to the ozone layer and have long been slathering themselves and their children with sunscreen. Many don't dare venture out between 11 a.m. and 3.30 p.m. in the summer – of course, this applies to everyone!

Some people, because of their skin type, have a much harder time in the sun than others and will never properly tan. Fair-skinned people can burn easily even if they take care – they must use a sun lotion with a high sun protection factor (SPF). Ask your pharmacist for advice on which lotions to use and you may escape the misery of sunburn!

Don't forget that in tropical countries and those close to the equator, the sun is much stronger and thus extra precautions must be taken. In the more intense heat you will need to take special care of the eyes and eyelids, lips, shoulders, breasts and tops of the feet. Limit your time spent in the sun, remembering that the early morning and the end of the afternoon is best. Apply sunscreen twenty minutes before you go outdoors, allowing it to be absorbed. Ten to twenty minutes of sun exposure on the first day is enough. Build up to thirty minutes gradually and always wear dark glasses and a large hat. Don't forget to drink plenty of water – your body will need to replace the liquid it has lost through sweating.

Too much sun can be extremely ageing to the skin. Under normal circumstances the skin will shed itself after exposure to the sun. This can be a gradual process and you may not even notice it. However, when you get sunburnt the process accelerates and more skin is shed, resulting in extra sensitivity. Many years spent sunbathing or using sunbeds on a regular basis, particularly if the skin is fair, will take its toll and cause early ageing. Deep wrinkles will appear, the skin will become excessively dry and it will begin to lose its elasticity (as the layers of collagen will be less evenly distributed). The skin will show irregularities in its colour and may even take on the appearance of leather!

Sensitive skins may gradually develop irregularities on delicate areas such as the face and particularly the nose. Keratoses can appear – these are small patches with brown, scaly surfaces. If you have them, ask your doctor to take a look as they can become more serious over time – red and sensitive. The same advice applies to moles, which also react to the sun. People with darker skins rarely suffer from keratoses as darker skins produce more melanin and thus have more resistance to harmful ultra-violet rays. Varicose veins and capillaries can appear in the sun too, as fragile capillaries expand in the heat, especially if you are lying prone and not moving.

Despite all the aforementioned precautions, the sun makes us feel so good and pampered and full of life, instantly putting us in a better mood. Our bodies need exposure to the sun to help make vitamin D and in small doses it is essential for our health and a good mental state. A dose of sunshine can instantly make a depressed person feel better and some dermatological conditions such as eczema, acne and psoriasis can benefit from sun exposure.

Essential oils and the sun

Essential oils and carrier oils should never be used directly in the sun. They can accelerate sunburn and growths. Bergamot, orange, grapefruit, lemongrass, lemon and lime are particularly contraindicated. Before going out into the sun, avoid face products that contain essential oils. However, some essential oils can help the skin to prepare for sun exposure. By massaging sensitive areas of your skin for a few weeks before a holiday, you can significantly reduce the risk of sunburn and prolong your tan.

Oil to prepare the skin before a holiday

This face and body oil should be applied to the skin for two weeks before a holiday. It should never be used in the sun as a protector, but can be applied after sunbathing (for instance, after a shower in the evening). This oil, with its high vitamin A and E content, will nourish your skin and give it suppleness and vitality. It will also reduce its sensitivity.

30ml (2 tablespoons) almond oil
30ml (2 tablespoons) avocado oil
20ml (2 dessert spoons) sesame oil
10ml (1 dessert spoon) argan oil
4 capsules wheatgerm oil
10 drops essential oil of carrot
4 drops essential oil of chamomile
4 drops essential oil of lavender
2 drops essential oil of rose
100ml bottle

Mix ingredients together. Shake well and massage into the skin at the end of each day. You can also add a tablespoonful of the oil to your bath. ❧

Another good way of preparing your skin is to drink carrot juice for a few weeks prior to a holiday. Take spirulina supplements and increase your intake of oily fish.

Avoiding holiday sunburn

Climate change means that the ozone layer is getting thinner and therefore we aren't as well protected as in the past from the sun's damaging ultra-violet rays. UVA rays are responsible for tanning the skin. These rays stimulate the melanocyte cells (in the lower layer of the epidermis) into producing melanin. Melanin acts as a natural protector, preventing the more serious UVB rays from getting to the cells. As the melanin disperses, the colour of the skin changes. If it is not dispersed evenly, the more harmful UVB rays can break through, causing freckles and burning. Your skin condition, age and skin tone are all significant factors in the production and distribution of melanin. You need to remember also that these harmful rays can penetrate the shade – even on cloudy days you are at risk.

If you are taking medication you should be very careful too, as some drugs can make your skin extra sensitive to the sun. Skin may react to ultra-violet rays quicker and sunburn can occur even in a short time. Consult your doctor about possible extra sensitivity because of any medication you may be taking.

If you have ever suffered from sunburn you will know that it can be incredibly painful. Burnt skin will become blistered, sore and tight.

Clothes can irritate the skin further and it can be impossible to sleep because of the discomfort. Sometimes in severe cases heatstroke can occur (see below).

Soothing lotion for sunburn with aloe vera

This soothing lotion is a wonderful way of rehydrating sunburnt skin.

1 cucumber
45 ml (3 tablespoons) aloe vera juice
2 drops essential oil of lavender
1 drop essential oil of carrot

Juice the cucumber and stir in the aloe vera juice, carrot and lavender oils. Mix well. Massage into the face and sunburnt areas until totally absorbed. Remove excess with warm water. Follow with an application of the nourishing face and body oil below. ❧

Nourishing face and body oil

20ml (2 dessert spoons) rose masqueta oil
20ml (2 dessert spoons) avocado oil
5ml (1 teaspoon) argan oil
4 capsules wheatgerm oil
5 drops essential oil of rose
3 drops essential oil of galbanum

Mix well and apply to skin after exposure to the sun. ❧

Cooling lavender treatment

A cooling tepid bath will really help sunburnt skin. Add five drops essential oil of lavender to running water and relax for up to ten minutes. Afterwards, put a few drops of neat essential oil of lavender on some cotton wool and apply to your sunburn. Next fill your washbasin with cold water, adding ten drops essential oil of lavender. Stir well. Plunge a T-shirt into it, wring, and then wear. A French doctor told me about this remedy twenty-five years ago and I have found that it is extremely soothing on sunburn – the T-shirt absorbs the heat from the skin and the lavender heals the skin.

It is important to stay out of the sun for a few days after sunburn, moisturizing your skin regularly in the mean time. Try this recipe: add five drops essential oil of lavender and two drops essential oil of carrot to a 50g pot of unperfumed, organic, moisturizing cream. Mix well and apply to your skin. ❧

Cooling spray for prickly heat and sunburn

When sweat glands become blocked due to sunburn, the tiny blisters and red spots of prickly heat will appear. It is terribly itchy, especially at night and can occur on all parts of the body.

1 sprig lavender or 1 head chamomile
600ml (1 pint) water
5 drops essential oil of eucalyptus
Spray bottle

Add your chosen herb to the water and bring to the boil. Let cool before pouring into the spray bottle and adding the eucalyptus oil. Spray on

affected areas. You can also place two cooled down chamomile tea bags on your eyes – an instant refresher! ❧

Cooling bath for sunburn and prickly heat

2 large tablespoons baking soda
3 drops essential oil of lavender

Mix well and add to running water. Relax for five to ten minutes. ❧

Chamomile lotion for prickly heat

Put two chamomile tea bags into a pan containing 600ml (1 pint) of water and bring to the boil. Leave to cool and use the lotion on cotton wool pads to calm itchiness. ❧

Heatstroke

Sometimes too much sun can cause headaches and dizziness; some people can feel nauseous. Put a drop of either essential oil of lavender, ravensare, geranium or peppermint on a tissue and inhale. Massage temples and nape of the neck with a little of your chosen oil. ❧

Faking it

I don't understand why so many people are happy to suffer in their quest for a tan when there are so many good fake tanning products on the market, which will help you achieve a good colour. If, however, you'd prefer to use a more natural product, try the suggestions here. A healthy glow can make you feel really good as people will comment on how well you look!

Natural fake tan

This wonderful recipe was given to me when I was in India. It is great for uplifting your skin colour.

Strong infusion of black tea
2 drops essential oil of rose

Add ten tea bags to a teapot and cover with boiling water. Infuse for half-an-hour to an hour. Add the essential oil of rose. Apply the lotion with a damp sponge, being careful around elbows, ankles and knees – you don't want a patchy effect!

Alternatively, you can make up a pot of very strong black tea – ten tea bags in a teapot. Infuse for fifteen minutes then add to running bath water with three drops essential oil of patchouli (this acts as a natural fixative, setting the colour). Make sure you fill the bath with enough water to immerse your whole body. Relax; check your elbows, knees and ankles periodically to make sure they're not patchy. Use a dark towel to dry yourself and one to stand on so you don't get the dark stained water on the floor. ❧

Jetlag

How can you take home lasting memories of a wonderful trip if you are plagued by jetlag, on the way out or on the way back? Flying off into the sunset is meant to be one of life's great pleasures but days (depending on time zones – one day per time zone according to my research) of unhappy recovery time is too much out of a short holiday. Most people experience some ill effects and symptoms of jetlag from flying long haul. Pressure from tight schedules, delays, cancellations, anxieties about take-off and landing, dehydration, sleep disturbance and general fatigue and weariness all seem to go hand-in-hand with long flights.

In the 1980s I started to think about all these awful symptoms and stresses, and after researching the subject I made myself up a special pack every time I flew long haul. Many fellow passengers were intrigued so I often shared my remedies with them!

The items I made myself included:

Eye compresses for tired and puffy eyes
Flower water used as a facial spray to combat dehydration
Some essential oils to help me sleep and others to wake me up
Nasal decongestive to help breathing
Ankle gel to massage into my ankles, boosting circulation

Essential oils can really help when travelling – after all, they are relaxing, calming, de-stressing and slightly hypnotic, easy to use and have wonderful scents too. Many of the preparations don't take long to make and they all have antiseptic and anti-bacterial properties – perfect protection against viruses. They also help to rebalance the body clock. Why not try and prepare your own basic essential oils travel pack before a long flight? It will certainly pay dividends.

Pampering travel pack

Rose or lavender flower water

This helps rehydrate the skin, which is important as many people suffer from dehydration when flying.

Add a few sprigs of fresh lavender or a handful of rose petals to 600ml (1 pint) of boiling water and leave to infuse. Once cool, strain and transfer 30ml (2 tablespoons) to a spray bottle and add one drop of essential oil of lavender or one drop essential oil of rose (depending on which flower water you've chosen). Shake well before use and spray on face when it feels dry. **Note:** Always close your eyes before spraying! ∿

Hydrating face oil

This face oil is extremely moisturizing and helps replace lost water. Choose between rose, chamomile, peppermint, lavender or ylang-ylang essential oils – you need just one drop.

Mix 10ml (1 dessert spoon) jojoba oil and one capsule of wheatgerm oil in a small bottle. Add one drop of your favourite essential oil and shake. When you're on the flight, massage the oil onto the face, neck and hands every two hours. ∿

Sleepy oil

Put ten drops essential oil of lavender and ten drops essential oil of petit grain into a small dark bottle. Add 5ml (1 teaspoon) of grapeseed or soya oil and a capsule of wheatgerm oil. Shake well. To relax and aid sleep, put a few drops on a tissue and inhale for a few minutes. Rub under nose

and sinus area, and on the nape of the neck. ∿

Wake-up oil

Put ten drops essential oil of rosemary and ten drops essential oil of juniper or geranium into a small bottle. Add 5ml (1 teaspoon) of grapeseed or soya oil and a capsule of wheatgerm oil. Shake well. For an instant pick-me-up, put a few drops on a tissue and inhale for a few minutes. Rub under nose and sinus area. ∿

Lip protector

For any length of flight, a lip protector balm is useful. Your lips are often the first area to suffer from the drying effect of cabin air.

½ teasoon of Manuka honey
3ml (½ teaspoon) aloe vera
5ml (1 teaspoon) castor oil or argan oil
1 capsule of wheatgerm oil
A few drops of freshly squeezed lemon juice
Jar

Mix the ingredients well in the jar. Apply several times during the flight. You can also use it several times a day if you suffer from cracked and dry lips. It will keep for up to two weeks in a cool place. ∿

More tips for coping with jetlag

Before you travel, there are lots of things you can do to reduce the effects of jetlag. You will be in a confined space on the plane so for a few weeks beforehand, start exercising your muscles – walking, jogging, swimming and aerobics are ideal.

Have a pampering massage before you go – petit grain, neroli, lavender, orange and melissa are all good. Make up an oil using two of the oils, five drops of each. Add the ten drops in total to a small bottle and add 30ml (2 tablespoons) of soya or grapeseed oil, and a capsule of wheatgerm oil. This will calm you down and help you relax. ᕰ

Arrive at the airport in good time so you don't get stressed. Once on the plane, try to make sure you get an aisle seat so you can get up and walk around easily – this is important as it will stretch the muscles and improve the circulation. Put a small suitcase or bag under your feet to elevate them, also improving circulation. Don't cross your legs and wear comfortable socks or slippers on your feet.

If you have enough space around you, massage or squeeze your feet from time to time (or get someone else to do it for you). Add three drops essential oil of geranium and three drops essential oil of cypress to 10ml (1 dessert spoon) of grapeseed oil in a small bottle. Use this to massage the feet and the ankles, repeating a few times. ᕰ

Remember to set your watch to the time of your destination so you can try to adapt straight away. Try to forget about the time at home!

Go easy on the alcohol as it will dehydrate and can be one of the biggest causes of jetlag. Drink a lot of water and don't eat too much – fruit is the best as it is easily digested. Avoid foods that will bloat your stomach and cause flatulence, such as broccoli, beans, cauliflower and peas.

The recycled, germ-filled air on planes is certainly not healthy, so take with you some essential oils with strong bactericide properties. In a small bottle, add five drops essential oil of eucalyptus and five drops essential oil of peppermint to 10ml (1 dessert spoon) grapeseed oil and a capsule of wheatgerm oil. Apply this oil inside your nose and on the torso from time to time. You can also inhale it to help the respiratory system. ᕰ

Half-an-hour before arrival at your destination, inhale some of your wake-up oil – place a few drops on a tissue or rub a little under your nose. Inhale deeply; rub the back of your neck, forehead and temples.

When you arrive at your destination, combat jetlag by trying to fit into the new time zone straight away – have breakfast if it's morning and if it's early and you're feeling tired energize yourself by adding a few drops of geranium or rosemary oils to a warm bath. Use the wake-up/sleepy oil for the first few days, inhaling when you're tired or need a pick-me-up. You could also put a few drops on your pillow.

Other travel tips

Peppermint inhalation for travel sickness

Place a few drops of essential oil of peppermint on a tissue and inhale to prevent and/or relieve symptoms. At your destination, add a few drops of oil to a bowl of hot water and place nearby. Peppermint tea will also help relieve symptoms of travel sickness. ᕰ

Insect bites and stings

Gently rub fresh lavender flowers or leaves onto the affected area. If not available, apply a drop of neat essential oil.

For wasp stings use neat essential oil of basil on a cotton bud or crushed basil leaves to calm the pain. ᕰ

Insect repellent

If diffused in a room, geranium essential oil makes a wonderful insect repellent. Add a few drops of essential oil to a bowl of hot water. You can also place a tissue, impregnated with the oil, beside your bed.

Add 30ml (2 tablespoons) of cooled-down boiled water to a spray bottle, followed by fifteen drops of essential oil of geranium. Shake well before use and spray the air around you, especially your bedroom at night. I always prepare a bottle to take with me on holiday, as there is nothing worse than the irritation of an insect bite! ᕰ

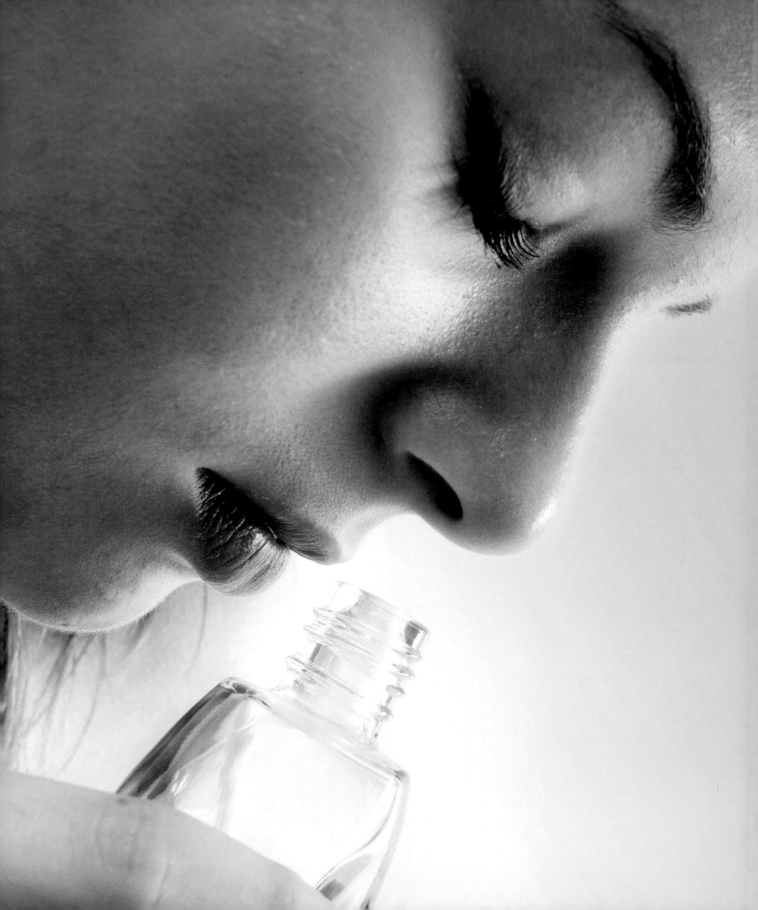

Creating your own perfume

Just mention the word 'perfume' to me and my well-trained nose will conjure up a beautiful, aromatic and therapeutic fragrance. But the image that usually springs to the minds of most people is a small, exquisitely cut, glass bottle – in other words, a distinctly average fragrance beautifully packaged by a designer brand. Today it seems that anyone can produce a perfume. It is the finishing touch to many a celebrity's portfolio and everyone seems to be doing it. I feel that much of the magic from the past has been lost in the wearing of perfume today. Fragrances that once held therapeutic and spiritual values are now too synthetic and intoxicating, many causing allergic reactions. There are too many bad perfumes on the market, mass-produced solely for the revenues they create.

Perfume through history

Perfume once held a strong place in society. It had a specific role to play in people's spiritual and physical lives, and different formulations were coveted and highly regarded. The word 'perfume' originates from the Latin for 'through smoke' and, in the past, fragrant resinous barks (cinnamon, benzoin etc.) were burnt as a way of cleansing and scenting the air. Many ancient civilizations used fragrances to communicate with each other, expressing their thoughts and emotions through smoke – a silent, scented correspondence.

The Japanese used aromatic substances to indicate the time and, at the beginning of every hour, a different fragrance was burnt – maybe a lighter scent in the morning followed by a heavier one at night. People told the time with their noses!

Ancient Egyptians burnt fragrances in order to please their gods – Horus, Isis and the sun god Râ. As the sun rose, the heady scent of burning sweet resins would fill the air, marking the start of the day. Prayers would be said in temples amongst the purified air and this ritual would be repeated at midday with the stronger scent of galbanum or myrrh. Hieroglyphics suggest that a combination of sixteen different fragrances (including frankincense) was burnt at night – a way of thanking the gods for the day.

The Egyptians gave their knowledge and skill to the Hebrew slaves. In the Book of Exodus, God told Moses to flee from Egypt and also advised him to take myrrh, cinnamon, olive oil and bulrushes to the New Land. These would help create a spiritual atmosphere in which to pray, enabling him to set up his temple.

It's wonderful that the Ancient Egyptians expressed themselves using different aromatic resins and barks. Also intriguing is the power of fragrances on the psyche – to aid prayer, concentration, meditation, spiritual healing. Therapeutic fragrances were given to worshippers as a means of elevating them to a higher state of consciousness. Inhalation of these perfumes was said to cleanse and rebalance the soul. It is also conceivable that the spiralling smoke was used as a communication device – a way of delivering messages to the gods.

When I was in India I noticed that some of the old temples were built with sandalwood. In the heat, the soothing, healing vapours penetrated me and I felt so spiritually connected. I was told that worshippers anoint their bodies with jasmine, rose, sandalwood and narcissus oils in preparation for prayer.

The Ancient Greeks used perfumes to protect themselves against diseases. They burnt fragrances in their homes as well as public places, so much so that the air in Athens became thick and polluted. As a result, Solon, one of the Seven Wise Men of Greece, introduced a law to ban their sale.

The word 'perfume' originates from the Latin for 'through smoke' and, in the past, fragrant resinous barks (cinnamon, benzoin etc.) were burnt as a way of cleansing and scenting the air.

The Romans adored certain fragrances and records show us that rose, especially Rose Gallica, was a particular favourite. On their travels, they filled the bottoms of their boats with rosebuds and became drunk on the scent. Old texts suggest that when Cleopatra first met Mark Antony, she ordered that the floor be strewn with rose petals, an inch deep. Wherever they walked, the fragrance was released.

The Romans brought a number of aromatic substances to the lands they conquered and continental Europe was quick to catch on. In France in the twelfth century, King Philip II Augustus encouraged local perfumers to exercise their skills, while in the court of King Louis XIV in the seventeenth century, people sprayed themselves with aromatic fragrances to mask bad body odours. The water was contaminated and full of diseases so washing with it was a definite no-no. It was during this time that Grasse became the world capital of the perfume industry and it still is to some extent nowadays although there is a lot less cultivation now than when it was at its height.

In England, perfumes were not really used greatly until the reign of Queen Elizabeth I. She received many gifts of perfume and would use them to scent her dresses, gloves and handkerchiefs. The ladies in her court were encouraged to make their own aromatic waters, pot pourri and scented linen. Many sewed little sachets of scented herbs into the hems of their skirts so the scent would be released when walking or dancing.

Perfume today

Perfume has thus played a role through many centuries and today the practice of making perfumes for pleasure has reached the peak of sophistication. A perfumer, known as 'the nose', has so many aromatic substances with which to work. There are over two thousand at his disposal and these can be mixed up into an infinite number of combinations – a skilled perfumer will be able to identify more than half of them by smell.

Some of these aromatic substances are derived from natural ingredients such as leaves, bark and flowers; others come from animal secretions (musk, civet and castoreum, but these are restricted today). Nowadays, however, price and availability mean that these natural ingredients are often substituted for synthetic versions.

A good perfume should make you feel young, well, uplifted, dynamized and boost your immune system. Unfortunately many of the chemicals that are used deliver a far from healthy punch. Recently I received a box of organic essential oils from France and it was truly one of my best gifts ever. After opening the bottles of jasmine, rose, neroli, ylang-ylang and others I was in a state of sheer bliss. Among them was a new lavender from Ukraine, which had an exquisite floral note. I felt incredible joy and it was a very pleasurable experience – how many shop-bought perfumes can do this?

Perfumes can evoke memories of people or places, or even be inspired by them. Guerlain expressed his love for a Japanese woman by creating 'Mitsouko', a heady scent with narcotic floral notes. 'Femme' by Rochas is spicy and sweet, and stirs up feelings of love.

Many women see perfume as an extension of their personality; it reinforces their image and some even use it to communicate. It can also be a master of mystery and can be used as a tool to mask fear and shyness. Too much, however, can be intoxicating and we must always be wary of the effect on others. A New York restaurant once banned the heavy floral perfume 'Giorgio' and I have moved seats in theatres before to get away from strong fragrances that have imposed on my sense of smell, making me feel nauseous.

Tips for perfume shopping

Interestingly, no perfume will smell the same on any two people. We all have our own body odours and these secretions and pheromones will intermingle with the different notes, making it unique to that individual. Be aware of this when you go perfume shopping. Don't do it in a hurry, have a positive attitude and don't attempt it if you're ill – the secretions emitted at this time will change the way the fragrance responds to your skin. Don't let the assistant behind the counter influence you – everyone has their own opinions. Try not to go shopping after eating spicy or garlicky food, as this can also alter your natural scent. Don't be tempted to wear your regular scent and hold back on strong body lotions too – they will clash. Avoid choosing a new perfume during your period as your sense of smell changes at this time (see page 96). Follow these tips and you won't make a costly mistake.

Spray the perfume on your wrist first, holding it out at a distance for a few seconds before you have your first smell. Never buy a bottle at this point, but allow the perfume to rise naturally and come back to it after a few hours. Ask for a sample or spray a little on a paper strip so you can smell it at a later stage. You don't have to stick with one perfume either, since moods can change, as do environments, and you may want a subtle scent for work and a more daring one for socializing.

The notes

Marguerite Maury once compared the notes of a perfume to those of music and the resonances of colour tones used by a painter. Just like a painter, a perfumer creates a special unique picture with aromas.

A perfume is composed of top, middle and base notes, with bridging fragrances in between. The top notes are light and are usually derived from more volatile substances such as citrus. These notes are responsible for the first impression. The heart of a perfume is made up of the middle notes. Released more slowly, these are typically rose or jasmine. Base notes are heavier and leave a lasting impression – sandalwood, oak moss, musk or frankincense, for instance. Lavender, palmarosa, bois de rose or geranium act as bridges, connecting all the notes together.

It's the interplay between these notes that creates a perfume's character. As the notes and aromatic substances resonate, the personality is revealed and the result can be heady, provocative, seductive, fresh or mischievous – there are so many possibilities!

Some good top notes for you to try: angelica, mandarin, lemon, petit grain, orange, lavender, chamomile, lime, peppermint, juniper, lemongrass, verbena, bergamot, basil, coriander, grapefruit, rosemary.

Here are some middle notes: jasmine, rose, tuberose, neroli, lavender, mimosa, marjoram, melissa, geranium, clary sage, clove, ginger, palmarosa, bois de rose, anise, ylang-ylang, violet leaves, thyme, iris, spikenard.

And some base notes: cinnamon, frankincense, myrrh, vetiver, sandalwood, galbanum, benzoin, patchouli, ciste.

Bridges and fixatives

Bridges and fixatives help to give the perfume tone and undertone, and link the notes together. It is like composing a piece of music. Good examples of bridges and fixatives include clary sage, vetiver, patchouli, sandalwood, mimosa, rose, galbanum, benzoin and bois de rose. Lavender is also good for light perfumes.

Remember that with some fragrances such as benzoin, they need to be warmed before the consistency is fluid enough to use. Place the bottle in a cup filled with hot water first and leave for a few moments before using. Mimosa is a sticky oil. If you would like to use it you will need to dissolve it in a little vodka or carrier oil first. Dip a cocktail stick into the mimosa oil and rotate between your fingers so the honey-like mimosa attaches itself to the stick. Dip the stick into an eggcup containing a small amount of vodka (2 teaspoons) or oil (2 teaspoons) to disperse. This represents about five drops.

Making your own perfume

Natural perfumes are gentler and not so detrimental to our health, as cloying synthetic perfumes can be. In fact they can be extremely beneficial to our health – Hippocrates said, 'Odoriferous molecules can influence a person's emotions, mental state … the way of life is through the essential oils of plants.'

Whenever you decide to make your own perfume ask yourself a few questions – what kind of impression would you like the perfume to give? How do you want to be perceived overall? Do you want to make a statement? Do you want to seduce or be seduced? How do you want the aromatic substances to smell – fruity, floral, woody or citrus? Do you want to recreate a memorable place or time? Would you prefer your perfume to have an alcohol or oil base? Don't forget that people will often notice your perfume before they notice other things and it is often the only thing that remains in a room after you've left. A good perfume will adorn you for ever and one that

Evaluating your perfume

❧ *Before you embark on making your own perfume you need to learn a little about each scent you have chosen, evaluating them one by one. This is a bit like meditation because you will need to visualize.*

Have a little notebook ready and place a drop of each essential oil in a bowl of boiling water. Stand at least half a metre away from the bowl otherwise you won't be able to pick up all the notes. Inhale the fragrance for a few moments.

Make a note of how it smells, is it:

Woody	*Green*	*Cold*
Herby	*Earthy*	*Light*
Leafy	*Warm*	*Heavy*
Floral		

You may also want to give your scents colours like red, pink, yellow, green, black, white, blue, grey. Familiarize yourself with each essential oil, day by day learning more. Take it in, inhale, relax and inhale again. Note your impression, write it down. Put a drop on a strip of blotting paper; after a couple of minutes inhale. (Remember to write the name of the oil on the back of the strip!) The next day do this with your eyes closed and try to remember the oil by its smell.

suits you can become more important than a favourite dress or piece of jewellery.

Decide if you'd prefer a stronger scent or a more subtle scent – an eau de toilette that you can spray on a few times during the day for instance. Choose between:

Perfume – very strong. For this you will need between 17–32% of pure fragrances to 90–95% alcohol (or oil).
Eau de parfum – this is 10–18% organic essential oils, 75–90% alcohol (or oil).
Eau de toilette – this is 6–10% organic essential oils to 70–75% alcohol (or oil).

The strength of your perfume will depend on the quality of your essential oils – you must use pure essential oils that have not been diluted or adulterated. It is difficult to buy pure alcohol so I have used vodka (make sure it's a strong proof!) with a little distilled water added. If you decide to go for the oil base there is no need to add water. Both oil and alcohol give quite different smells as the molecules expand in different ways with time.

Use a notebook to record all your ingredients carefully. It is essential that you do this as every drop counts – if you add one too many or one too few you can completely change the composition (remember one drop represents approximately 500g–1kg of flowers). It is important to be methodical and disciplined and soon you'll be able to make bespoke perfumes for your family and friends.

You can have lots of fun too – buy a pretty cut glass bottle, making sure the top fits properly. Bespoke perfumes like these need to 'cure' before you first use them – keep them in a cool dark place for between four to six weeks so the ingredients have a chance to blend together properly and the molecules have time to expand.

If you find the fragrance too strong, add a little more vodka and water to make it into an eau de toilette. If you choose an oil, add a little more grapeseed oil. You will also need to add a natural fixative (these are also bridging oils) – clary sage is a good oil to use for this.

Note: I've used eau de parfum in my examples because this is the most popular version. Home made perfumes should keep for six months to a year.

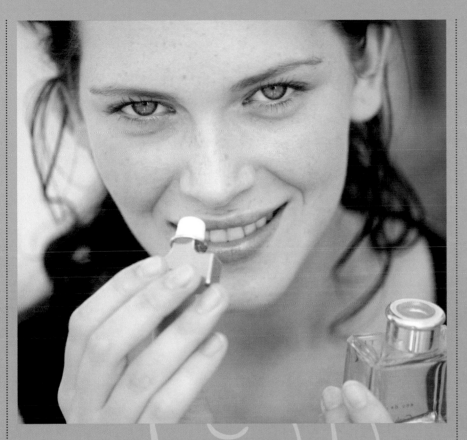

Example eau de parfum in oil

This gives a gentle scent; if you'd like to make it stronger, add more drops in the top and middle notes.

Top notes
20 drops essential oil of orange
15 drops essential oil of petit grain
15 drops essential oil of lavender

Bridge I
5 drops essential oil of either
*   palmarosa or benzoin*

Middle notes
20 drops essential oil of neroli
25 drops essential oil of rose
20 drops essential oil of either bois
*   de rose or violet leaves*

Bridge II
5 drops essential oil of clary sage
Base notes
15 drops essential oil of galbanum
15 drops essential oil of either
*   sandalwood or cedarwood*

50ml jojoba oil
30ml (2 tablespoons) grapeseed oil
4 capsules wheatgerm oil
100ml bottle
1 coffee filter

Pour the carrier oils into the dark bottle first and shake well. Add the essential oils, working from the base notes upwards as before. Shake once and leave to 'cure' before first use (see page 162). Strain through a coffee filter before transferring to a nice bottle. ✌

Example eau de parfum in alcohol

I want this to have a nice citrus smell, so if you'd prefer a heavier scent, increase the drops of the base-note oils.

Top notes
20 drops essential oil of lemon
10 drops essential oil of either
*   bergamot or bois de rose*
20 drops essential oil of petit grain

Bridge I
5 drops essential oil of lavender

Middle notes
15 drops essential oil of either gera-
*   nium or ylang-ylang*
25 drops essential oil of either
*   jasmine or tuberose*

Bridge II
5 drops essential oil of clary sage (this
*   will also be your fixative)*

Base notes
10 drops essential oil of vetiver
8 drops essential oil of sandalwood

70ml vodka
5ml (1 teaspoon) distilled water
100ml bottle

Add the water and the vodka to the dark bottle followed by the oils. Start with the base-note oils first, bridging II oils and work upwards to the top notes. Shake once and leave to 'cure' (mature) before first use (see page 162). Transfer to your nice bottle. ✌

Bibliography

Many of my sources of reference are research papers and books published in other languages such as French or German, which have not been translated into English, thus the titles for these are given in French or German.

Dr Belaiche, *Classification des Huiles Essentielles en Fonction de leur Pouvoir Antiseptique Guide Familial, La Médicine par les Plantes* (Hachette 1982)

Jean Claude Bourret, *Le Defi de la Medecine par les Plantes* (editions France Empire 1978)

C. Cadeac et A. Meunier, *Traveaux Divers, Comptes Rendus Socio-biology* (1889)

F. Caujolle et C. Frank, *Sur les Proprietes des Huiles Essentielles* (1945)

A. Couvreur, *Plante à Parfum et Plantes Aromatiques* (1930)

Dr F.J. Cazin, *Traite Pratique et Raisonne des Plantes Medicinales* (1876)

Department of Agriculture, New South Wales, Australia *Tea Tree Oil* (1989)

Dr Delioux de Savignac, 'Essence de Mente Analgesiante' (*Therapeutic Journal*, 1875)

Pierre Franchomme, *La Science de L'Aromatherapie, Encyclopedie sous la Direction Scientifique* (2003)

Paul Faure, *Parfums et Aromates de l 'Antiquité* (Fayard 1987)

Dr René Maurice Gattefossé, *Antiseptiques Essentials* (Desforges, Giradot et Cie 1931)
Distillation des Plantes Aromatiques et Parfums (1926)
Le Pouvoir Bactericide des Essences (1919)

Maud Grieves, *A Modern Herbal* (Jonathan Cape 1979)

Dr G. Guibourt, *Histoire Naturelle des Drogues Simples* (1876)

Hippocrates, *History of Health and Medicine* (Pelican 1978)

Dr Leclerc, *Precis de Phytotherapie* (Masson et cie 1969)

Dr A. Maury, *La Médecine par le Vin* (Edition Antulen 1988)

Marguerite Maury, *Le Capital Jeunesse* (1961)
The Secret of Life and Youth (Macdonald & Co. Publishers Ltd 1964)
Marguerite Maury's Guide to Aromatherapy (C.W. Daniel 1989)

Eugene Perrot, *Matieres Premieres Usuelles du Regne Vegetal* (1940)
Les Plantes Medicinales (1970)

Dr Pomet, *History of Drugs* (1694)

G. Rattray Taylor *The Science of Life* (A Panther Book 1963)

R. Rideal et A. Walker, *Le Pouvoir Bactericide de Chaque Essence Aromatique* (1930)

A. Rouviere et M.C. Meyer, *La Sante par les Huiles Essentielles* (MA Edition 1938)

Danièle Ryman, *Danièle Ryman's Aromatherapy Bible* (Piatkus 2002)
Aromatherapy Hand Book (Century Publishing 1984)
Aromatherapy in Your Diet (Piatkus 1996)

Dr Jean Valnet, *Docteur Nature* (Editions Fayard 1980)
Phytotherapie et Aromatherapie (Presses de la Renaissance 1978)
Aromatherapie Traitement des Maladies par les Essences de Plantes (Maloine 1964)

F.V. Wells and M. Billot, *Perfumery Technology* (Ellis Horwood Publications 1975)

V.A. Worwood, *Aromatics* (Pan Books 1978)

For further information

For recommended sources of where to obtain essential oils and carrier oils, information on courses, lectures on aromatherapy and industry updates, please refer to

www.danieleryman.com

Index